Indirect Procedures

Indirect Procedures

A Musician's Guide to the Alexander Technique

Pedro de Alcantara

CLARENDON PRESS · OXFORD

1997

Oxford University Press, Great Clarendon Street, Oxford OX2 6DP
Oxford New York
Athens Auckland Bangkok Bogota Bombay
Buenos Aires Calcutta Cape Town Dar es Salaam
Delhi Florence Hong Kong Istanbul Karachi
Kuala Lumpur Madras Madrid Melbourne
Mexico City Nairobi Paris Singapore
Taipei Tokyo Toronto
and associated companies in
Berlin Ibadan

Oxford is a trade mark of Oxford University Press

Published in the United States
by Oxford University Press Inc., New York

British Library Cataloguing in Publication Data
Data available

Library of Congress Cataloging in Publication Data
Alcantara, Pedro de, 1958–
    Indirect procedures : a musician's guide to the Alexander
  Technique / Pedro de Alcantara.
      p.   cm.
    Includes bibliographical references and index
      1. Musicians—Health and hygiene.   2. Alexander technique
    RC965.P46A43   1997   615.8'2—dc20   96–19690
        ISBN 0–19–816568–4
        ISBN 0–19–816569–2 (pbk)

10 9 8 7 6 5 4 3 2 1

Typeset by Graphicraft Typesetters Ltd., Hong Kong
Printed in Great Britain
on acid-free paper by
Biddles Ltd.,
Guildford & Kings Lynn

To the memory of Patrick Macdonald

Acknowledgements

To compose, which comes from Latin, only means to place together. I like to think that I did not write this book so much as compose it. Some readers may accuse me of having done a cut-and-paste job. Others, I hope, will think that I have some powers of synthesis which mitigate my lack of originality. For I do not say anything in this book that has not been said before, usually in a manner more compelling and elegant than mine, and I thank the men and women whose insights have guided and nourished me. (I lifted the first line in this paragraph from a clever and beautiful song by Red Mitchell.)

I owe all I know about the Alexander Technique to my teachers, the late Patrick Macdonald and Shoshana Kaminitz. Mr Macdonald did more than anyone else to preserve and further Alexander's discoveries. A man of fierce integrity, Mr Macdonald had a fabulous nonsense detector, and would undoubtedly object to much of my writing. I appreciated Mr Macdonald's straightforward manner and his sense of humour. I think of him every day of my life, with gratitude and pride. Shoshana Kaminitz is a marvellously imaginative, skilful, and dedicated teacher. Without her help my understanding of Mr Macdonald's teachings would be woefully inadequate.

I thank my cello teachers: Barney Lehrer, Robert Gardner, Daniel Morganstern, Aldo Parisot, and William Pleeth. May they recognize their presence in the book and forgive me for having dismembered them for my wicked purposes. I thank some of my other teachers, whose presence also permeate this book: Joan Panetti, Jenny Kallick, Harold Samuel, and Otto-Werner Mueller. I thank my first singing teacher, the late Roy Hickman, and my beloved mentor, Robert D. Levin.

I thank readers of early drafts of parts of the book: Adam Nott, Alex Farkhas, Orlando Murrin, Antonia del Mar, James Johnson, and others. I always lapped up their compliments, but sometimes ignored their criticisms, proving that I am vain and stubborn. All the faults of this book belong therefore exclusively to me.

Some years ago I received a generous grant from FAPESP, a research foundation run by the state of São Paulo, Brazil. The grant entailed my writing a thesis about the Alexander Technique and music-making, which became the basis for this book.

I thank Marjorie Hodge. In her mind's eye she saw the writer in me much earlier than I saw him myself, and I cherish her encouragement and support.

Finally, I thank my pupils. Carl Rogers, the great American psychologist, went to Brazil some years ago for a series of workshops and conferences, at the end of which he announced that he learned more from his students than his students from him, and refunded his fees forthwith. (The Brazilians found this scandalous.) Had I Rogers's integrity, I would have to pay my pupils to take lessons from me. I thank them for their commitment and patience, as well as for paying me in cash all these years.

Illustrations

Fig. 1: photo by Chris Joyce for Rover Cars, courtesy of Rover Cars (with thanks to Nikki Rowlinson of LINTAS*i*); Fig. 2: from *Joys and Sorrows, by Pablo Casals as told to Albert H. Kahn* (New York: Simon and Schuster, 1970), by kind permission of Mrs Albert H. Kahn; Fig. 3: photo of cellist Janos Starker, courtesy of Colbert Artists Management, Inc., New York, NY; Fig. 4: © David Redfern/Redferns, by permission; Figs. 5 and 14: from Herbert R. Axelrod, ed., *Heifetz* (Neptune City, NJ: Paganiniana Publications, 1976), by kind permission of Dr Axelrod (with thanks to David Zarowin); Fig. 6: photo by Martha Swope, © TIME Inc., by permission; Fig. 7: by kind permission of Linda Lee; Fig. 8: by kind permission of Walter Vaughan-Jones; Fig. 9: courtesy of the Furtwängler Archives, Zentralbibliothek, Zürich (with thanks to Chris Walton); Fig. 10: © Eugene Cook, by kind permission of Phyllis Curtin (with thanks to Martine Bailly); Figs. 11, 15, and 16: © Rosangela Mesquita, by kind permission (with warm thanks to Ms Mesquita, Jodi Forrest, and Georgina Peacock); Fig. 12: © The Board of Trustees of the Victoria & Albert Museum, by permission (with thanks to Shoshana Kaminitz); Fig. 13: by kind permission of Michel Harmon; Fig. 17: courtesy of the Rubinstein family (with thanks to Eva Rubinstein); Fig. 18: © Eva Rubinstein, by permission; Fig. 19: by kind permission of Christian Tissier; Fig. 20: photo by Cate Novas, by kind permission of Christian Tissier; Fig. 21: by kind permission, Biddulph Recordings (with thanks to Jim Johnson); Fig. 22: courtesy of the Primrose International Viola Archive (with thanks to Prof. David Dalton); Fig. 23: © STAT, by permission.

Grateful acknowledgement is made for permission to reprint excerpts from the following copyrighted works:

Extracts from F. Matthias Alexander's *Man's Supreme Inheritance*; *The Universal Constant in Living*; and *Articles and Lectures*: by permission of the Estate of F. Matthias Alexander © 1996. Extracts from F. Matthias Alexander's *Constructive Conscious Control of the Individual* and *The Use of the Self*: by permission of Victor Gollancz.

Wilhelm Furtwängler, *Notebooks 1924–1954*, translated by Shaun Whiteside (London: Quartet Books, 1989): by kind permission of the publisher. Tito Gobbi (with Ida Cook), *My Life* (London: Macdonald and Jane's, 1979): by kind permission of Rupert Crew Ltd. Margaret E. Hogg, *A Biology of Man*, vol. 2, *Man the Animal* (London: Heinemann Educational Books, 1966): by kind permission of Heinemann Educational, a division of Reed Educational and Professional Publishing Ltd. Frank Pierce Jones, *Body Awareness in Action: A Study of the Alexander Technique*, with an Introduction by J. McVicker Hunt (New York: Schocken Books, 1976): by kind permission of the Jones family. Bruce Lee, *The Tao of Jeet Kune Do* (Santa Clarita, Calif.: Ohara Publications, Inc., 1975), © copyright 1975 by Linda Lee: reprinted by kind permission of the publisher. Patrick Macdonald, *The Alexander Technique as I See It* (Brighton: Rahula Books, 1989): by permission of the publisher. Bruno Monsaingeon, *Mademoiselle: Conversations with Nadia Boulanger*, translated by Robyn Marsack (Manchester: Carcanet Press, 1985): by kind permission of the publisher. Heinrich Neuhaus, *The Art of Piano Playing*, translated by K. A. Leibovitch (London: Barrie and Jenkins, 1973): by kind permission of the publisher. Oliver Sacks, *The Man who Mistook his Wife for a Hat and Other Clinical Tales* (New York: Harper Perennial, 1990): by kind permission of the author, c/o Rogers, Coleridge & White, in association with International Creative Management. Nancy Toff, *The Flute Book* (London: David & Charles, 1985): by kind permission of the publisher. Peter Wingate, with Richard Wingate, *The Penguin Medical Encyclopedia*, 3rd ed. (London: Penguin Books, 1988): by kind permission of Peters Fraser & Dunlop Group Ltd. W. B. Yeats, *A Dialogue of Self and Soul*: in the United States, its territories and dependencies, and the Philipine Republic: reprinted with the permission of Simon & Schuster from THE POEMS OF W. B. YEATS: A NEW EDITION, edited by Richard J. Finneran, copyright 1983 by Macmillan Publishing

Company, copyright renewed © 1961 by Bertha Georgia Yeats; in the rest of the world, reprinted from the Collected Poems of W. B. Yeats by permission of A. P. Watt Ltd on behalf of Michael Yeats.

Warmest thanks to Cornelius L. Reid for his permission to quote from his books, *The Free Voice: A Guide to Natural Singing* (New York: Joseph Patelson Music House, 1972); *A Dictionary of Vocal Terminology: An Analysis* (New York: Patelson Music House, 1983); and *Essays on the Nature of Singing* (Huntsville, Tex.: Recital Publications, 1992).

The author was unable to trace the copyright holders of *Singing: the Physical Nature of the Vocal Organ. A guide to the unlocking of the singing voice*, by Frederick Husler and Yvonne Rodd-Marling (London: Faber and Faber Ltd., 1965).

Foreword

SIR COLIN DAVIS

> It is what man does that brings the wrong thing about, first with himself and then in his activities in the outside world; it is only by preventing this 'doing' that he can ever begin to make any real change.
>
> F. M. ALEXANDER

Many people now have heard of the Alexander Technique, and know that F. M. Alexander dreamed of the restoration of 'good use of the self'. So how and when did we lose this 'good use' we were born with and enjoyed as infants? On the journey. Yeats has said it for us: we must all

> Endure that toil of growing up;
> The ignominy of boyhood; the distress
> Of boyhood changing into man;
> The unfinished man and his pain
> Brought face to face with his own clumsiness;
>
> The finished man among his enemies?—
> How in the name of Heaven can he escape
> That defiling and disfigured shape
> The mirror of malicious eyes
> Casts upon his eyes until at last
> He thinks that shape must be his shape?
>
> (from 'A Dialogue of Self and Soul')

Can one find the way back, restore that 'good use' and the other things that went with it, and re-win through the longest journey the ability to live again as a small child? I do not know: but I do think it worth the effort. Work on that 'disfigured shape', strive to restore it, strip away the varnish—that obscuring sediment of the years of conflict between the attempt to think well of oneself and the deepening knowledge of one's inadequacy for the task!

Alexander's 'way' was a real discovery: he found another means to confront the old problem of the mechanical man, slave to his idea of himself. His teaching gives us a new interest in ourselves. The attention of a good teacher makes us—as Mozart makes us—for all our absurdities, acceptable to ourselves. It helps us to be aware of useless habits and petrified opinions, and to accept the possibility of change, however small, therefore progressing along the 'way' and escaping the perpetual threat of becoming that inert pillar of salt which is Death in Life.

I shall always remain grateful to Sir Adrian Boult, who sent me to Wilfred Barlow for my first Alexander lesson. 'My boy!' he said, 'you'll be a cripple if you go on like that!' That was some forty years ago. Now my wife is an Alexander teacher herself and our family of musicians takes lessons from her. It is clear that we are all convinced of the importance of the Technique. It is not a cure, it is not exercise, it is not analysis, but it does involve working upon oneself in every aspect of one's behaviour, and comparing the freedom attained through the lesson with one's shackled progress throughout the day, while here and there an echo may reach us of 'the hidden laughter / of children in the foliage'.

'Be careful of the printed matter,' said F. M. Alexander. Yes, but what else have we? And how could we read between the lines were no lines there? Persevere! There is much wisdom here in this book, along with some great quotations, many photographs, and exhaustive analyses of the aims and applications of Alexander's discoveries. If there is one phrase or one sentence that suddenly speaks to the reader and sets his or her foot upon the way, then Mr Pedro de Alcantara's huge effort is more than justified. Take some lessons and *bon voyage!*

Preface

It is quite difficult for the average reader to learn geology or trigonometry from a textbook, without the help of a qualified and sympathetic teacher. With subjects in which sensorial experiences are an integral part of the learning processes, it becomes impossible to learn directly from a book. Many good books have been written about singing, for instance, but nobody expects to learn how to sing from reading them. Similarly with the Alexander Technique. This book is not a do-it-yourself manual. It is meant as a guide to people who have studied the Alexander Technique or who are studying it now. It is also meant to awaken the curiosity of readers who have never had an Alexander lesson; I sincerely hope that such readers will go on to take lessons in the Technique—the only way of learning it. Throughout the book I shall remind all readers repeatedly of the impossibility of understanding sensorial experiences through the written word; I apologize to those who find my insistence upon this point tiresome.

Throughout the book I refer to generic Alexander teachers in the third person feminine, and generic pupils in the masculine. This is not to say that all teachers are women—I, for one, am a man, unless I am mistaken. The same observation applies to the use of the masculine pronoun, and to the use of the word 'man', by which I mean 'a human being'.

Contents

List of Illustrations

Abbreviations

All books are by Frederick Matthias Alexander.

AL *Articles and Lectures*, with a foreword by Walter H. M. Carrington and notes by Jean M. O. Fischer (London: Mouritz, 1995)

CC *Constructive Conscious Control of the Individual*, 1923 facsimile of the 1st edn. (Downing, Calif.: Centerline Press, 1985)

MSI *Man's Supreme Inheritance*, 1910 (London: Chatterson Ltd., 1946)

RB *The Resurrection of the Body: The Essential Writings of F. Matthias Alexander*, selected and with an introduction by Edward Maisel (New York: Dell Publishing Company, 1974)

UCL *The Universal Constant in Living*, 1941, facsimile of the 1st edn. (Long Beach, Calif.: Centerline Press, 1986)

US *The Use of the Self*, 1932 (Kent: Integral Press, 1955)

Introduction

A child prodigy who once played like an angel loses his innocence and becomes self-conscious about his instrument, his music-making, his adoring public. Despite much soul-searching, he is unable to prevent his performances from becoming ever more erratic.

A young man, one of the outstanding talents of his generation, suffers from disabling back pain, due, it seems, to a birth defect. He needs major back surgery while still in his early twenties. His enormous success with the public and the critics notwithstanding, some of his fellow musicians—who have followed closely the blossoming of his exquisite gift—find some of his performances strangely dissatisfying.

A young woman of flair and ability is marketed by her record company as a classical-music sex kitten. She admits to having developed three distinct personalities—with her family, on stage, and by herself—to cope with the expectations and demands made upon her.

A magazine survey shows that an alarmingly large majority of orchestral musicians live in a state of constant apprehension and insecurity. Many of them drink heavily before and after performances, and during the intervals as well. Others take tranquillizers and anxiety-suppressants. Most complain of various illnesses seemingly related to work, including backaches, headaches, tendonitis, repetitive strain injuries, ulcers, and a plethora of mental conditions, including depression and plain unhappiness.

The behaviour of many eminent conductors, singers, and soloists deviates sharply from accepted standards of human decency. The temper tantrums, cancelled performances, and generally outrageous comportment of the diva make the stuff of gossip columns. We are told that these are a necessary evil, a sign of an 'artistic temperament'.

The waste of talent, the shortened careers, the inadequate performances, the objectionable behaviour, the frustration, suffering, and pain are the norm of the music profession. Yet one asks, 'Must it be so?' Is there something intrinsic to music-making that makes it inevitably painful?

The answer, of course, is no. We marvel at the effortless grace of Artur Rubinstein, at the high quality of his every performance, at his youthfulness in old age. We listen, enraptured, to the mastery of a Vlado Perlemuter, a Richter, a Perahia. We revere a Claudio Arrau, whose playing had the depth and breath of a wise old man and the dazzling virtuosity of a young competition winner. We take inspiration from great singers who remain great for decades, and who perform, teach, and live with quiet dignity.

Musicians of all ages and abilities, faced by seemingly insurmountable problems, have offered many good reasons for their shortcomings and failures. Yet, in light of the successes of other musicians, these reasons don't stand up to scrutiny.

A well-worn explanation for the troubles of a musician—and, indeed, of everyone else—is stress. In *Anatomy of an Illness as Perceived by the Patient*, Norman Cousins wrote that 'the most prevalent—and, for all we know, most serious—health problem of our time is stress, which is defined by Hans Seyle, dean of the stress concept, as the "rate of wear and tear in the human body." This definition would thus embrace any demands, whether emotional or physical, beyond the ready capability of any given individual.'[1]

This very definition of stress is wide of the mark. Let us borrow an image from engineering. We say of a bridge that it is under *stress* (from the constant traffic flow, for instance, or from the action of the elements) and that it, the bridge, *strains*. The bridge suffers wear and tear and may crack or collapse as the result—not of stress, but of strain. Stress is a stimulus, strain a response. Clearly it is the response that causes a problem, not the stimulus; after all, many bridges have withstood centuries of unremitting stress. The stress of life is permanent and inevitable, and in itself it is neither negative nor undesirable. Witness the many healthy musicians who thrive under the most stressful situations, including baring their souls in front of hundreds or thousands of people.

A related argument is that of 'human design'. You may argue that well-built bridges withstand stress, but that the human body was not designed to bear what is made to bear today. This is a double fallacy: of 'human design' and 'modern civilization'.

Let us consider human design first. Many people believe that a small body was not meant to play the viola, or that a small hand was not meant to play the piano, or that the human voice was not designed to sing above modern symphony orchestras. This argument runs a long way. We were not designed to run marathons, to wear shoes, to walk on concrete, and so on.

Yet the argued insufficiency or inadequacy of human design is easily disproved. 'For playing the viola,' said the violist and teacher William Primrose, 'having a large hand and being of medium to large stature is an advantage, but certainly not a requirement.'[2] The pianist Heinrich Neuhaus, teacher of Sviatoslav Richter, Emil Gilels, and Radu Lupu, among many others, went further, and wrote in *The Art of Piano Playing*:

The anatomy of the human hand is . . . ideal from the point of view of the pianist and it is a convenient, suitable and intelligent mechanism which provides a wealth of possibilities for extracting the most varied tones out of a piano. And the mechanism of the hand is, of course, in complete harmony with the mechanism of the keyboard.[3]

Small hands with a small stretch have quite obviously to make much greater use of wrist, forearm and shoulder; in fact the whole of the 'hinterland', than large hands, particularly large hands with a large stretch. . . . Sometimes this is just why gifted people with small and difficult hands have a better understanding of the nature of the piano and of their 'pianistic' body, than the large-handed and broad-boned. . . . *In short, they turn their drawbacks into advantages.*[4]

Let us abandon the 'human design' fallacy and agree with Hamlet that humans are 'the beauty of the world, the paragon of animals', fully evolved bipeds with lovely opposable thumbs and countless other attributes. The human body, wondrously beautiful and richly endowed, is capable of meeting all the demands of music-making.

'Human design apart,' you may argue, 'progress has led us so far from Nature that humans are now constitutionally unable to cope with the demands of modern civilization. Take orchestra chairs, for instance. *They* are badly designed. Or music competitions. Surely they are harmful. What about going on long tours? Living in big cities? Breathing in car exhaust? Life was better before. If only we could give up the rat race and move to the countryside. Or go back to the eighteenth century. Or the sixteenth. Or just return to Eden.'

Thus runs the 'modern civilization' argument. The intentions behind it are noble, but the argument itself is flawed.

Some observers, for instance, find chairs emblematic of the ills of modern life. They say that if only an ideal chair could be built, many health problems would be mitigated or eliminated. In Shakespeare's *All's Well that Ends Well*, the Clown speaks a few lines that help us recognize the limits of ergonomics: 'It is like a barber's chair, that fits all buttocks,—the pin-buttock, the quatch-buttock, the brawn-buttock, or any buttock.'[5] Such a chair will never exist. Further, no furniture, however designed, can give you health if you do not know how to use it. Badly designed furniture increases the likelihood of discomfort, well designed furniture decreases it; no certitudes arise of either. 'What we need to do', wrote Alexander, 'is not to educate our school furniture but to educate our children.'[6]

Competitions are another scourge of the anti-civilization brigade. It is said that competitions have poisoned the music profession, destroyed the careers of young musicians, and perverted the tastes of the public. In truth competitiveness is a healthy, irrepressible human instinct, and every culture at every junction of history has had a competitive element. Would music be better served had the great singers of the Bel Canto era not been pitted against each other in competition? Should Wales outlaw its Eisteddfodau?

Realistically, we cannot blame competitions themselves for the woes of any musician, young or old, winner or loser. It is the attitude of the competitor that makes competitions either beneficial or harmful. Rod Laver, the great Australian tennis champion, said about competing:

You do the best you can. If you don't play your own game, you're going to lose it anyway. If you start to worry about the importance of the win before it happens, you're going to have yourself in a complete panic. You play the shots as you see them. That, and don't start wishing the shots to go in. When you start wishing, you are in trouble.[7]

As I noted, the logical consequence of blaming modern life for our problems is to wish to go back in time, a sneaking desire we all feel on occasion. Indeed, people already felt that way thousands of years ago. 'Say not thou, What is the cause that the former days were better than these? for thou dost not enquire wisely concerning this.' Beautifully written in Ecclesiastes, this advice can also be stated as 'Yearning for the past is stupid.' If our capabilities to meet life's demands are inadequate, then we need to increase our capabilities, rather than decrease the demands made upon them. The right way clearly is forwards, not backwards.

Another favoured cause for a musician's problems is *other people*. Some would argue that pushy parents, or pushy record executives, caused the young woman of my illustration to suffer from split personality. Orchestral musicians blame conductors and administrators for their woes. Conductors and administrators blame orchestral musicians and each other. Singers blame everybody.

Stress, human design, civilization, and other people, then, have all been considered part of a musician's problems, and appropriate therapies suggest themselves. Pushy parents cause psychological problems; the solution is psychotherapy. Small hands cause tendonitis; the solution, physiotherapy. Bad chairs cause backache; the solution, ergonomics. The stress of concert life causes stage fright; the solution, beta-blockers. Modern life causes unhappiness; the solution, a return to Nature.

These solutions have been around for a long time, and have been tried by many sufferers. Yet the problems persist. If anything, the overall situation of the music profession is worse today than it was one or two generations ago. Disability and grief have increased, excellence has decreased.

A diagnosis always implies a remedy. Get the diagnosis wrong, and the remedy may threaten the patient's life. We can safely say that the way in which musicians diagnose their problems has become part of the problems themselves. Psychotherapy, physiotherapy, drugs, and the rest have failed to solve the problems of musicians satisfactorily.

Frederick Matthias Alexander (1869–1955) understood the nature of human ills and proposed effective solutions, not palliatives or aggravations to these ills. As I wrote earlier, Alexander considered most of contemporary thinking fallacious. He thought that we erred both in the diagnosis and in the therapy. Alexander found the cause of our troubles not in what is done to us, but in what we do to ourselves. He saw that the problem was not in the stimulation of modern life, but in our response to it; not in the stress, but in the straining. The straining he called *misuse of the self*; its cause not human design, but *end-gaining*. I shall explain both terms and their relationship in the next chapter.

The advantages of Alexander's approach are manifold. Alexander found the common thread to apparently disparate problems. Instead of saying that pushy parents cause neuroses, Alexander stated that end-gaining causes misuse. He would not say that bad chairs cause backache; again, he would suggest that end-gaining causes misuse. He would similarly reformulate the equation between body design and tendonitis, civilization and stress, and all the others.

Alexander's discoveries offer both a diagnosis and a remedy, thereby unifying the whole of the equation: End-gaining causes misuse; the solution, inhibition—a concept which I discuss in Chapter 4. Thus is the Alexander Technique able to solve more problems, and more efficiently, than the piecemeal approaches of psychotherapy, physiotherapy, surgery, drugs, ergonomics, and firing the conductor.

Part I
The Principles

1 *The Use of the Self*

Unity of Life

One of the great clichés of our time is that Man is indivisible, his body, mind, and spirit inseparably interwoven. The dichotomies of body and mind, of reason and emotion, of objectiveness and subjectiveness, of God and Man that once shaped the theories and practices of Western life are no more. Today we see things differently: Descartes is out, Lao Tse in. Man is one not only within himself, he is also one with the Universe. And that is why we eat brown sugar instead of white. For this is the extent to which most people incorporate the new, holistic thinking in their daily lives.

'A vision of the world that is merely talked about, i.e. one to which lip-service is paid, which is at best *known*, rather than one that is lived and active, is the signature of our contemporary conditions.'[1] Wilhelm Furtwängler wrote these words two generations ago, but today they are more urgent than ever. The ghosts of Descartes and Augustine still haunt us. The old dichotomies remain; all we did was to subvert their underlying moral judgements. It used to be: mind good, body bad. Reason good, emotion bad. Authority good, free will bad. Today we say: body good, mind bad. Feeling good, thinking bad. Free will (self-expression, spontaneity, individuality) good, authority (hierarchy, discipline, control) bad.

Medicine sees mind as largely detached from body. As Dr Oliver Sacks wrote, 'a split [has] occurred, into a soulless neurology and a bodiless psychology.'[2] We admire an athlete's body and a university professor's mind. Symptomatic of this dichotomy is that we see the workings of the body as separate from the behaviour of the body's owner. 'My shoulders are tight,' we say; or, 'I have a weak back,' not 'I'm tightening my shoulders,' not 'I misuse my back.' We see the workings of the mind too as separate from the behaviour of the mind's owner. He beats his wife, he cannot change a light bulb, he is smoking himself to death, but he won a Nobel prize. 'What *brains*!'

Musicians think along the same lines. Off the top of our heads we define 'technique' (such as violin technique) as 'the physical means to actualize a musical conception'. (In Chapter 15, 'Technique', I shall argue that this is a limited and limiting definition.) A violin teacher writes of stage fright as having physical, mental, or social causes. (Pigeon-holing the causes of stage fright, she sets up compartmentalized solutions as well.)

'The formal dichotomy of the individual [into "body" and "mind"],' wrote the biologist Sir Charles Sherrington, '. . . which our description practised for the sake of analysis, results in artefacts such as are not in Nature.'[3] Language both reflects and shapes the way we think. Say 'body' and, naturally enough, you will think of 'the body', a separate entity with a life of its own—an artefact such as is not in Nature. To free ourselves of the belief that such an entity exists, we need to free ourselves of our very language.

Alexander was a far-sighted man, and his genius is manifest not only in his theories and practices, but in his vocabulary as well. On the one hand, he relied on little technical jargon; a glossary of the Technique would not have more than a half-dozen terms. On the other hand, he refrained from using words which imply a separation of body and mind, like 'body mechanics' and 'mental states'. Instead, he spoke simply of 'the self' and its use and functioning.

Sir Charles Sherrington wrote compellingly about the self and its unity. His words constitute a proper definition of the term:

Each waking day is a stage dominated for good or ill, in comedy, farce or tragedy, by a *dramatis persona*, the 'self.' And so it will be until the curtain drops. The self is a unity. The continuity of its presence in time, sometimes hardly broken by sleep, its inalienable 'interiority' in (sensual) space, its consistency of viewpoint, the privacy of its experience, combine to give it status as a unique existence. Although multiple aspects characterize it it has self-cohesion. It regards itself as one, others treat it as one. It is addressed as one, by a name to which it answers. The Law and the State schedule it as one. It and they identify it with a body which is considered by it and them to belong to it integrally. In short, unchallenged and unargued convictions assume it to be one. The logic of grammar endorses this by a pronoun in the singular. All its diversity is merged in oneness.[4]

Alexander did not divide the self into body and mind; further, he did not subdivide the mind. In practice this means that for Alexander the body did not control the mind (or vice versa); neither did the 'subconscious' control the 'conscious' (or vice versa). He explained that his own conception of the 'subconscious self' 'is rather of the unity than the diversity of life. [In connection with the expression "conscious control"], this conception does not necessarily imply any distinction between the thing controlled and the control itself.'[5]

This is a pointer to Alexander's understanding of how the self works. It invalidates the common metaphor of the body as a car, and the brain as its driver. I shall discuss this issue further in the next chapter.

The Use of the Self

Alexander often wrote of the self as something 'in use', which 'functions' and which 'reacts.' He entitled one of his books *The Use of the Self*, and we can say unequivocally that the Alexander Technique is not a method of physical relaxation, or posture, or the use of the body, but of the use of the self. Alexander again:

When I employ the word 'use,' it is not in that limited sense of the use of any specific part, as, for instance, when we speak of the use of an arm or the use of a leg, but in a much wider and more comprehensive sense applying to the working of the organism in general. For I recognize that the use of any specific part such as the arm or leg involves of necessity bringing into action the different psycho-physical mechanisms of the organism, this concerted activity bringing about the use of the specific part.[6]

I should like to give an example. Imagine yourself talking with a person you know. The subject-matter is unimportant; so is the identity of your friend. In this situation both of you are speaking. Each voice has its timbre, colour, resonance, diction, and inflection. Both of you use your vocal mechanisms, lips, tongue, jaw, the breathing apparatus, and the whole body besides. Each of you has a personal choice of words, grammar, points of view, and ways of arguing them. You swear, or not; you stammer, stutter, whisper, shout, laugh, or not. You gesticulate; you laugh by throwing your head back; you interrupt your friend. Your friend lisps and drools. You are loud, brash, unreasonable, angry. Your friend is timid, hesitant, unclear; he looks away when he addresses you.

At no point during your discussion would it be possible for you to say that speaking is a purely physical act, or purely mental. The way you use your voice is a concerted activity of your entire self. It would be better to refer not to the way you *use your voice*, but the way you *use yourself while speaking*, thereby acknowledging the completeness of this act. This use of the self is unique to you, and indivisible in its multiple manifestations.

Let us draw a few conclusions from our hypothetical situation.

1. *The part reflects the whole.* The use of your voice reflects the use of your whole self: it reflects *who you are*. Further, the use of each part of your voice (vocabulary, intonation, gesticulation) also reflects the use of your whole self. Indeed, your every activity engages your whole self, and is representative of your uniqueness. I recognize your voice from a single 'hello' on the phone. An iridologist draws deep insight about your well-being from examining your irises, a reflexologist from handling your feet, an acupuncturist from taking your pulse—proof positive that the part always reflects the whole.

2. *Every part of the self always plays a role, regardless of the situation.* If when I speak I do not move my arms at all, their passiveness is one of the defining characteristics of my use. The term 'use' does not imply activity: to let my arms stay still is a way of using them. In every situation many parts *should* play a passive role, this being an important element in the co-ordinating of the whole self, and one which I address throughout the book.

3. *Every part is always connected to every other part.* My diction and my vocabulary are connected to the timbre and resonance of my voice. The use of my voice is linked to the use of my arms, and vice versa. The use of my arms is connected to the use of my neck, shoulders, and back.

The use of the self, then, is the way I react, with the whole of myself, in any given situation. Alexander put it succinctly: 'Talk about a man's individuality and character: it's the way he uses himself.'[7] The self does not consist of two halves (body and mind) or three thirds (body, mind, and spirit) that work together; it consists of a whole, so unified in its workings that no separate part (body, mind, spirit) can be said to exist independently of the others.

If you do accept that you are whole and indivisible, you will need to speak differently, to think differently, to practise, rehearse, and perform differently, to heal your diseases differently. For if you *are* one, you *work* as one, and you cannot examine, change, or control one of your parts separately from the whole.

Intelligence and Posture

Two observations may help you understand the self not as body and mind combined, but a single entity that always works as a whole. These observations concern 'intelligence'—the workings of the mind—and 'posture'—the workings of the body.

Defining intelligence is a matter of some difficulty. A scholar who writes clearly and elegantly on an important subject can behave in inadequate and unhealthy ways. Is he intelligent? In a discussion of artificial intelligence, Professor Michael Brady, of Oxford University, states that the ability to reason or think 'is not what intelligence evolved for. I think sensing and action—not thinking—are the very well-spring of intelligence'.[8] An intelligent man is one who acts and lives intelligently—a man who uses himself well. 'When I speak of the "knowledge" of an artist,' wrote Heinrich Neuhaus, 'I have always in mind an active force: understanding plus action. Or simpler still: acting correctly on the basis of correct thinking.'[9]

For the convinced Alexandrian, 'thinking' refers not to a purely intellectual activity, but to an activity of the self in living. According to this view, correct thinking always leads to correct acting, and correct acting always ensues from correct thinking. Indeed, the two are inseparable.

The Technique is often associated in the public mind with posture. Posture is not synonymous with use, but it is certainly one of its elements. Some Alexander teachers have said that the Technique concerns itself with *postural behaviour*, a concept which encompasses posture and goes beyond it.

Generally we understand posture as a bodily position we hold, consciously or unconsciously, for some length of time. Now that we agree that body and mind are inseparable, we must alter this definition. Talk of 'good posture' to an unsuspecting friend, and he will immediately 'straighten his back', push his shoulders back, and hold himself rigidly, in an imitation of a stereotypical soldier or a bad dancer. He does not realize that posture (the visible arrangement of bodily parts) is inextricably linked to a set of attitudes, thoughts, and feelings. Indeed, posture is tantamount to attitude.

Posture and movement also are more closely linked than generally believed. The biologist George Coghill knew Alexander and supported his work. Of posture he wrote:

In deep sleep [a condition illustrative of immobility] the individual is mobilized in regard to its visceral, circular and respiratory functions and the like. . . . The distinction between mobility and immobility is relative, and no absolute distinction can be made between them. . . . [Under the circumstances of mobility] the organism is in one of two phases of action, posture or movement. . . . In posture the individual is mobilized (integrated) for movement according to a definite pattern and in movement that pattern is being executed. [The differences between posture and movement] are relative, and one phase passes over imperceptibly into the other. . . . In posture the individual is as truly active as in movement.[10]

In short, there is nothing to separate posture from attitude, nor from movement. To define posture as a bodily position is then doubly misleading.

Alexander and other teachers, notably Patrick Macdonald, wrote clearly on the subject of bodily positions. Alexander's argument is simple. Human growth is never-ending, and each individual develops in a unique way. If you could find a 'right position', it would be right for you only, and for a short period of time. My right is of necessity your wrong, and your right of today your wrong of tomorrow. 'There is no such thing as a right position, but there is such a thing as a right direction,' said Alexander.[11] This will become clearer after our discussions of the Primary Control, in the next chapter, and of direction, in Chapter 5.

Enlightened musicians understand the fallacy of looking for a fixed position. 'I maintain that the best position of the hand on the keyboard is one which can be altered with the maximum of ease and speed,'[12] wrote Heinrich Neuhaus. This applies equally to hand positions at the instrument and to 'positions of the body', or posture.

Tension and Relaxation

Neuhaus says that good positions can be altered with ease and speed. Many musicians would conclude that what they need to ensure such ease is physical relaxation. However, there are two faulty assumptions in this conclusion. One is that so-called physical relaxation can exist independently of the workings of the mind. It might be better to speak of relaxation without the attached qualifier. This is not simply semantics; the way you define relaxation will shape the way you pursue it.

The second assumption—that relaxation is indeed desirable—

deserves close scrutiny. 'Pupils sometimes mistake the concept of "favourable position," "convenience," for the concept of "inertia" [i.e. relaxation],' wrote Neuhaus. 'These are not only two entirely different things, they are also contradictory. The attention required for ensuring well-ordered, organized playing, . . . excludes both physical and spiritual inertia.'[13]

True relaxation, illustrated by the apparent effortlessness of Rubinstein or Heifetz, is not the cause of a musician's mastery of his instrument, but an effect of it. It is, therefore, useless to seek out relaxation in itself. Giovanni Battista Lamperti wrote in his book *Vocal Wisdom*:

Relaxing a muscle is beneficial only to educate and discipline outermost muscles to do their part in the process.

Otherwise it is weakening to the final output.

It is co-action, not non-action, that causes controlled effort to feel effortless.

. . . Singing is accomplished by opposing motions and the measured balance between them.

This causes the delusive apearance of rest and fixity—even of relaxation.[14]

The singing voice in reality is born of the clash of opposing principles, the tension of conflicting forces, brought to an equilibrium.[15]

The word 'tension' has acquired an unwarranted negative connotation. When somebody complains of tension, he really means too much tension, or, more precisely, the wrong *kind* and *amount* of tension, in the wrong *places*, for the wrong *length of time*. In itself tension is not negative. 'Tension is a proper adjunct of human behaviour—one cannot live without it,'[16] wrote Patrick Macdonald. Tension creates and sustains life, and carries it forwards. Tension—of the right kind—is a prerequisite of dynamic, energetic, vital human endeavour.

The cause of wrong tension is most often the lack of right tension. In such cases it is fruitless to try to relax these wrong tensions directly; the solution lies in creating the right tensions, and letting relaxation come about on its own. Consider a pianist who stiffens his neck, shoulders, and arms when playing. It is likely that he tenses his neck simply to compensate for a lack of *necessary tension* elsewhere. If he uses his back and legs to support his shoulders and arms properly, then his neck will relax itself—an instance of an indirect procedure.

The importance of this issue and the magnitude of the misconceptions attaching to it merit another illustration. The singing teacher Cornelius L. Reid writes:

All visible, external signs of effort reflect a condition in which muscles are relaxed when they should be in tension. If the muscles of the laryngeal and pharyngeal tract are not properly engaged, the energy used in singing must be directed elsewhere and, as a consequence, the muscles of the jaw, neck, shoulders, and chest will come into tension when they should be relaxed. These muscles can only be made to relax, however, when the coordinative process is reversed. Successful reversal of a faulty technique will cause interfering tensions to disappear without their ever having been made a matter of direct concern.[17]

I argued earlier that the Alexander Technique is not a method of bodily positions, as there are no right positions, only right directions. I maintain now that the Technique is not a method of physical relaxation either. Good use of the self entails *right tension*—right in type, amount, placing, and timing. I shall give further thought to the questions of positions, directions, tension, and relaxation throughout the book.

Use and Functioning

When I first described how we conceive of body and mind as separate, I pointed out that we also see the workings of the self as separate from the self itself. If I say, 'My back is weak,' I assume somehow that the state of my back does not have much to do with me. This is me, and that is my back, which gives me trouble.

Alexander's genius consisted in disproving this assumption. If a human being is truly one and whole, then surely there is no distinction between 'the thing controlled and the control itself'. It is a simple but revolutionary understanding of how we work. It is not my back that gives me trouble, but I who give it trouble. The way I use myself affects the way I function, and to improve my functioning *I must change my use.*

To appreciate better the relationship of use to functioning let us consider a number of situations where this relationship is subverted.

1. *Singing in the mask.* A singing teacher asks her pupil to sing in the mask, or to 'bring the tone forwards'. (The mask is the facial area around the nose and eyes. Behind it lie cavities which some singing teachers believe to be the main resonators of vocal tone.) A singer who

sings in a certain way may subjectively feel as if she were placing her tone forwards. Frederick Husler and Yvonne Rodd-Marling write that, useful fiction that this may be, 'the sounding of a resonating chamber [in this case the so-called mask] is always a *secondary* manifestation, the result of muscle movements in the vocal mechanism. . . . It goes without saying that the *first* causes for the various *acoustic* phenomena that occur in singing lie in the vocal organ itself, and it is these that the voice trainer must learn to hear.'[18] In other words, the sounding of a resonating chamber is an aspect of the *functioning* of the singing voice, and the muscle movements in the vocal mechanism constitute its *use*. To affect the functioning of the voice the singer has no choice but to act upon its use; therefore, to try to place the tone forwards directly is a patent absurdity. Unfortunately most teaching directives of mainstream, contemporary singing pedagogy are based on attempts to affect functioning, not use. This is the case with both 'support' and 'breath control', which I shall discuss in Chapter 8, 'Breathing'.

2. *Diagnosing backache.* A trombonist has backache. His doctor diagnoses a weak back, and recommends a programme of weightlifting and swimming. Yet consider this: on the one hand, top athletes—men and women of towering strength—suffer from back trouble like everyone else. On the other hand, an old African woman can carry immense loads easily balanced on top of her head, without ever injuring herself. She has no more muscular strength than an athlete or than our troubled trombonist. Surely the trombonist's problem is not weakness but misuse. Strength is the result of good use: an effect, not a cause: 'I am strong *because* I use myself well'—and not 'I use myself well because I am strong.'

3. *Conducting.* An orchestral conductor conceives an interpretation in his mind's ears. The music as he imagines it awakens certain emotional and bodily responses in him. Then, much as a child marches enthusiastically to martial music, the conductor choreographs his bodily reactions to his conception of the piece, in the hope that the orchestra will reproduce the sounds that made him react this way in the first place. Yet an orchestra cannot possibly become a cause to the effect that the conductor choreographs. The harder the conductor tries to make the orchestra obey his will the worse it plays. Soon the conductor throws one of the temper tantrums for which he is feared the world over. The orchestra sounds no better at the end of the rehearsal. Conducting is not unlike horseback riding. Mary Wanless writes in *Ride with your mind*:

The rider can have far more influence on the horse than I had ever imagined possible. Often, when I was riding a horse who seemed rigid and unyielding, a better rider would take over, and I would watch the horse transform before my very eyes, becoming far more beautiful in his movement, more proud in his carriage, and more *willing* in his demeanour. It was as if the rider was a sculptor, and the horse was his material: when I rode him he was completely inflexible, but in the hands of one of these good riders he became a malleable medium, ready to be moulded into whatever shape and movements the rider chose for him.[19]

The better rider does not scream at her horse or whip him, nor does she tighten her legs on the horse's back to make him obey. Rather, she uses herself well, and the horse responds accordingly. Every aspect of a conductor's use affects the performance of an orchestra. Like a horse under different riders, an orchestra changes almost miraculously under different conductors, thanks in good part to the differences in their use. I repeat Alexander's words: 'Talk about a man's individuality and character: it's the way he uses himself.' If a conductor wishes to affect the functioning of the orchestra, all he needs to do is to make changes in his own use, rather than trying to control functioning directly.

End-Gaining

In the Introduction I wrote of Alexander's understanding of cause and effect. When somebody complains of a weak back, Alexander speaks of misuse of the self. When an orchestral musician blames badly designed chairs for his fatigue, Alexander speaks of misuse of the self. When a conductor faults an orchestra for a bad performance, Alexander speaks again of misuse of the self.

To solve these problems, it would seem enough to stop the misuse of the self. However, the chain of cause and effect goes further. It is only logical to ask, 'What *causes* misuse?' Most people would readily blame education, civilization, modern life, family life, religion, or the lack of religion. Alexander believed otherwise, having realized that the problem lies not in what is done to you, but in what you do to yourself. Faced with the constant stimulation of life, you can react healthily—using the best means any situation requires—or unhealthily—achieving your ends with disregard to the best means whereby your end may be achieved. The ultimate cause of misuse, in Alexander's understanding, is the universal habit of *end-gaining*. This is at the core of the Technique, and we need some clarifying examples.

1. End-gaining is both a concept and a procedure. To diagnose the back pains of our trombonist as the result of a weak back is already to end-gain, even before any action is taken. This diagnosis looks at an end result, not its cause, namely misuse of the self. The suggested remedy, swimming, is an end-gaining remedy. In and of itself swimming will not eliminate misuse. And the trombonist in the swimming pool becomes a water-borne end-gainer. He swims by trial and error, in a manner dictated by instinctive guidance and control and concerned mostly with getting to the other side of the pool. He misuses himself when he swims, and his back hurts after a swim as much as it does after a rehearsal or performance.

2. The father who screams at a child for her to stop crying is end-gaining. The means he uses achieve the opposite end from the one he desires. Likewise the conductor and the seemingly disobedient orchestra. In truth the out-of-control orchestra reflects faithfully the out-of-control conductor, and cannot therefore be called disobedient.

3. The singer who attempts to bypass use and to control functioning directly is an end-gainer. She goes directly to her ends—the sounding of a resonating chamber, the economy of breath, the beauty of the tone—thereby neglecting the means whereby she can achieve these ends.

4. The young musician intent on winning a competition is an end-gainer. Alexander recounts the following anecdote, about a match involving W. H. (Bunny) Austin at Wimbledon:

At one stage in the game, [Austin] was playing so badly he decided not to try to win the set but . . . as soon as he had made that decision, he began to play up to his usual form. In consequence, he decided that now he would try to win the set after all, and immediately reverted to the indifferent play that had caused him 'not to try.' It does seem sometimes as if human beings not only like to be fooled by others but are keen on fooling themselves.[20]

Simply put, to go directly for an end (to win) causes a misuse of the self (the indifferent play) which makes the end unattainable. Enter competitions, then, wishing not to win but to do your best, which may or may not assure you of a prize.

The list of examples could go on for ever. End-gaining is the most prevalent of all habits. It is so widespread and insidious that most people do not realize that they, and others, are end-gaining all the time. To take your shoes off without untying the laces (thereby ruining their heels) is to end-gain. To drive a car on the hard shoulder of a clogged road is to end-gain. Weight-loss diets are end-gaining; a healthy diet helps you attain your ideal weight, but a weight-loss diet is usually unhealthy. It is end-gaining to take medicaments with the sole purpose of suppressing symptoms of disease. To blame others for the results of your own actions is to end-gain. To try to change others rather than to change yourself is to end-gain.

In an Alexander lesson, the teacher helps you to become aware of your end-gaining in simple acts of daily life, such as sitting, standing, walking, speaking, using your arms, and so on. As you become aware of each *instance* of end-gaining, you become aware of end-gaining *itself*, and with time your understanding of end-gaining should encompass everything you do.

The 'Means-whereby' Principle

The antithesis of the end-gaining principle is called the 'means-whereby' principle. Simply put, it calls for you to create and use the best possible means to achieve any given end. This involves the ability to wait and to make reasoned choices before acting, the awareness of your own use at all times, and the willingness to give up achieving your ends by direct means (such as yelling at a child to stop her crying). Indeed, the means-whereby principle is but an *indirect procedure*.

Frank Pierce Jones, an Alexander teacher, gave an interesting definition of the means-whereby principle in the glossary of his book, *Body Awareness in Action*:

Means-whereby—The co-ordinated series of intermediate steps which must be accomplished in order to attain an end. The means-whereby principle is the recognition in practice that these intermediate steps are important as ends in themselves, and that the most important step at any time is the *next* one. Application of the means-whereby principle involves awareness of the conditions present, a reasoned consideration of their causes, inhibition of habitual or end-gaining responses to these conditions, and consciously guided performance of the indirect series of steps required to gain the end.[21]

I disagree with one item in this definition. In a series of intermediate steps, the most important step at any time surely is the one being performed at that very moment, the next step being the second most important. Imagine that there are five steps to the execution of an exercise. If, for instance, you are going through the performance of the second step, it and it alone should be foremost in your mind—not the previous step, not the outcome of the combined steps, not the end you want to achieve.

The means-whereby principle applies to all situations: diagnosing and solving problems, practising, rehearsing, and performing, executing simple actions or perfecting complex skills. I shall explain and illustrate the principle throughout the book.

Use and Habit

The self being an indivisible unit, the use of its every part affects the use of the whole. You may well ask, 'If I decide that some aspect of my use needs improving—the use of my right wrist at the piano, for instance—do I have to effect changes to *all* other aspects of my use? It would take me for ever to achieve what I want.'

The way you use your wrists at the piano is but a habit. Like all habits, it is a familiar reaction to a certain stimulus. You may have developed it consciously or subconsciously, and you may be aware of it or not. The habit may be harmful or not.

A habit only becomes a problem when it is automatic, harmful, and beyond the control of the conscious will. Imagine a pianist who consistently misuses his wrists. He suffers from incipient pain; his passage-work is uneven and his sound small. For him, his misuse is both a habit and a problem.

To appreciate how the Alexander Technique achieves specific results without disregarding the fundamental unity of the self, let us consider Alexander's definition of habit:

The influence of the manner of use is a *constant* one upon the general functioning of the organism in every reaction and during every moment of life, and . . . this influence can be a harmful or a beneficial one. . . . From this there is not any escape. Hence this influence can be said to be a *universal constant in a technique for living*.[22]

'Habit, indeed,' wrote Alexander, '*may be defined as the manifestation of a constant*.'[23] The pianist's use of his wrists is a habit, and as such it is the manifestation of a constant: the influence of use upon functioning.

This has extremely practical consequences. Since the influence of use upon functioning is a constant, changing use causes an inevitable *indirect* change in habit (a manifestation of this constant). Rather than controlling habit by acting upon it *directly*, work on your use instead.

A Case History

I should like to illustrate this point with a case history. Joanna is an accomplished concert pianist and teacher who sought the help of the Alexander Technique after she was diagnosed as suffering from carpal tunnel syndrome, a painful condition of the wrist. I quote *The Penguin Medical Encyclopedia*:

carpal tunnel. A fibrous bridge, the *flexor retinaculum*, spans the small bones at the base of the palm of the hand. The carpal tunnel is the opening between the flexor retinaculum and the bones. The flexor tendons to the fingers pass through this tunnel, enclosed in slippery synovial sheaths which prevent friction in this narrow space. Between the tendons is the *median* nerve.

The *carpal tunnel syndrome* arises from compression of the median nerve in the tunnel. In the hand, the median nerve carries motor fibres to the muscles of the ball of the thumb and sensory fibres from the thumb and the index, middle, and ring fingers. Pressure on the nerve causes pins-and-needles, numbness, or pain in this area, and sometimes weakness of the thumb. Arthritis or injury of the wrist may produce this syndrome, but usually there is no obvious reason for it. The fact that it is commonest in middle-aged women and during pregnancy suggests a glandular disturbance. The symptoms are often worse after lying down. Some cases respond to splinting the wrist at night. Injection of hydrocortisone usually gives at least temporary relief. If these simple measures fail, the condition is often cured by cutting the constricting fibres of the retinaculum.[24]

Untreated, this condition leads to permanent disability. Medical diagnosis today is supplemented by the view that this condition may be caused by overuse of the wrist; carpal tunnel syndrome is a specific instance of a repetitive strain injury (RSI). Medicine offers the choices of rest, physiotherapy, cortisone injections, and surgery.

Alexander teachers propose a different approach. Carpal tunnel syndrome is not caused by over-use of the wrists, but by misuse—of the whole self, including the wrists. To rest the hands would not be a solution; if the misuse persists, the problem will recur after the period of inaction. Wrist exercises based on the end-gaining principle risk becoming part of the problem, not the solution. Cortisone (which alleviates the pain without altering the condition itself) is an extremely powerful drug with serious side-effects. Surgery does not address the problem of misuse; some operations are indeed life-saving, but others are unnecessary and maybe even harmful.

Joanna's wrist problem was symptomatic of a larger picture. In everything that she did, at the piano and away from it, she misused her whole self. She habitually contracted her head into her spine, twisted her trunk, shortened, narrowed, and curved her back, lifted her shoulders, and created excessive tension in all her limbs.

Her use (her 'individuality and character') had other defining characteristics. Joanna was a volatile woman who reacted quickly and strongly to whatever happened around her. Her speech was often agitated and suffused with sentiment. In effect, she always over-reacted, and her interpersonal relationships were marked by needless antagonism. Joanna, like many people today, was addicted to stimulation of all sorts: intellectual, emotional, sensorial, gastronomic. She ate extremely quickly, consumed large amounts of sugar and chocolate, had digestive problems, and was several pounds over her ideal weight.

She was a talented and well-trained pianist, technically proficient, musically sophisticated, and comfortable in front of an audience. She was bright, imaginative, and enterprising. Her misuse was not more pronounced than other people's, but it was catching up with her and causing pain—as it usually does, sooner or later, in the average person.

Her painful wrist was a by-product of her whole way of being—the manifestation of a constant. The only way of ridding herself of this manifestation was to change the underlying constant. For an Alexander teacher to 'treat her wrist' and leave everything else untouched would be unthinkable. Yet it would be equally preposterous to work on her habits of speech, digestion, interpersonal relationships, piano playing, and so on. As habits, these are all manifestations of the same constant.

Joanna's misuse exerted a constant harmful influence upon her functioning. Obviously the solution to her problems lay in her stopping her misuse. By using herself well, she would reverse this harmful influence upon her functioning; in due course her good use would exert a constant, beneficial influence upon her functioning, including that of the wrist.

Besides demonstrating the relationship between use and functioning, Alexander showed that there exists a certain mechanism of the head, neck, and back that affects the *total* use of the self. He called this the Primary Control, and I shall describe it in the next chapter.

My work with Joanna consisted largely of helping her change the use of her Primary Control, according to the principles and procedures outlined in this book. We did not address her problematic wrist directly. Neither did we work on her speech, her dietary habits, or her piano playing. And yet, over a period of time, she started eating differently and losing weight. She presented herself more elegantly. She became considerably less reactive, without losing her ability to react. She reported finding new and, to her, startling colours at the piano. She changed her piano teaching, which was dominated by pedagogical formulas and by the drive for quick results. She became less antagonistic in her relationships. Her newly found co-ordination helped her have a trouble-free pregnancy. Her mountain climbing, one of her hobbies, became easier. She effected positive changes in every one of her habits—of work, food, love, and play.

Needless to say, she saved her wrist from a risky operation and from cortisone injections of dubious value, and she saved herself from early retirement as a pianist. The Alexander Technique does not cure illness. Rather, it aims to change the constant influence of use upon functioning, thereby changing all manifestations of this constant. If Joanna starts end-gaining again, her pain may well return. Next time around, however, she may look upon her pain simply as a reminder of her duties to herself.

2 The Primary Control

A Case History

Mark, a cellist, plays for me in a lesson. I notice that when he plays he tends to look intently at his left hand. Presumably he thinks that he can control his hand better by looking at it. But since there are no frets in a cello, looking at his hand will not guarantee precise intonation. Further, I am sure that, were he to play in a darkened room, he would still look at his hand, as if he could actually see it. In short, his looking at his hand is a permanent habit based on an end-gaining idea of controlling visually something that he should control kinaesthetically (that is, by muscular feel).

By looking at his left hand, Mark triggers a pattern of total misuse of the self. He twists his head and contracts his neck, thereby tightening his shoulders, torso, and left arm. Tension spreads to his right arm and both legs as well.

This misuse affects his functioning. Mark's sound is scratchy at the heel of the bow and feeble at the tip. His intonation is faulty, his vibrato constricted, and his left-hand changes of position are unreliable. His breathing is agitated and noisy. Mark tires easily and suffers from stage fright. His back hurts, and his left wrist shows signs of tendonitis.

Alexander discovered a mechanism that regulates the workings of the use of the whole self. This mechanism involves the relationship of the head to the neck, and of the head and neck to the back. Alexander called this relationship the *Primary Control*. Mark's problems, which are characteristic of an average musician, demonstrate both how use affects functioning and how the Primary Control governs total coordination.

The biologist George Coghill wrote in an introduction to one of Alexander's books:

In my study of the development of locomotion I have found that in vertebrates the locomotor function involves two patterns: a total pattern which establishes the gait; and partial patterns (reflexes) which act with reference to the surface on which locomotion occurs.

... Now the reflexes may be, and naturally are, in harmony with the total pattern, in which case they facilitate the mechanism of the total pattern (gait), or they by force of habit become more or less antagonistic to it. In the latter case they make for inefficiency in locomotion.

... Mr. Alexander, by relieving this conflict between the total pattern, which is hereditary and innate, and the reflex mechanisms which are individually cultivated, conserves the energies of the nervous system and by so doing corrects not only postural difficulties but also many other pathological conditions that are not ordinarily recognized as postural.[1]

The Primary Control is that 'mechanism of the total pattern' in the use of the self. Ideally the total pattern (hereditary and innate, in Coghill's words) should take precedence over all the partial patterns (individually cultivated). In other words, every localized action—the activity of limbs, hands, and fingers, and of lips, tongue, and jaw—should be executed in harmony with the co-ordination of the head, neck, and back. Mark pays undue attention to a partial pattern, the use of his left hand. In the process he distorts his total pattern, the use of his head, neck, and back. The resulting misuse affects every part of his organism, from head to toes, and every aspect of his functioning, from vibrato, intonation, and shifting to sound-production, breathing, and general well-being.

Characteristics of the Primary Control

Like other discoveries that depart from accepted wisdom, the Primary Control is easily misunderstood. It would be useful for us to consider what the Primary Control is *not*.

1. *Naturalness and artificiality*. It is not something you *acquire*; everybody who is born with a head, a neck, and a back already has a Primary Control. What you may acquire, develop, and refine, however, is a certain way of using your Primary Control. Learning a conscious use of the Primary Control may 'feel new' to you, but this is not to say that it is artificially contrived. Since healthy children, well-co-ordinated adults, and wild and domesticated animals use their Primary Control in this way, we can only call it *natural*—according to the laws of Nature. Looking at an average, badly co-ordinated civilized man it

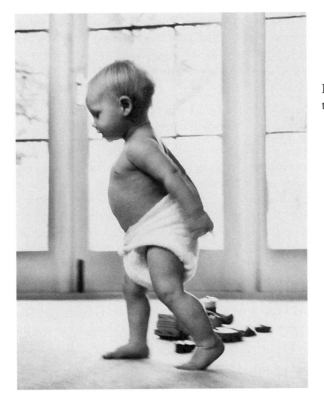

FIG. 1. The head leads,
the body follows

is difficult to appreciate the importance of the Primary Control and
the beauty of its workings. But watch a cat jumping, or a gazelle running, and you can see clearly how the orientation of the head influences the organization of the whole organism. In human beings the
Primary Control may manifest itself differently—a biped will necessarily use his head and neck differently from a quadruped—but it has
the same integrating effect on total co-ordination. In humans as well
as in animals, 'the head leads, the body follows.' This is beautifully illustrated by the picture of the infant learning to walk (Fig. 1).

2. *Unity of the self.* The Primary Control is not something your
'body' does independently of your 'mind'. Physiology has given us an
accurate explanation of the way the Primary Control works on one
level, but this is not to say that it works on that level alone. Here is a
partial description of its mechanical workings:

The most important proprioceptive impulses [in the maintenance of balance and
in space orientation] arise in sense organs located within the muscles themselves
and in the joints and tendons. These proprioceptors inform the nervous system

of the position of the limbs relative to the rest of the body; a sagging joint or a drooping head both cause changes in angles and pressures at the joints and stretching of the muscles.... [The] stimulation [of the proprioceptors] sets in train a type of reaction known as a stretch reflex: it is upon such stretch reflexes that the so-called tone in the muscles is basically dependent.[2]

The proprioceptors in the muscles ... are called muscle spindles.... Closely associated with each spindle is the branch end of a sensory nerve fibre ... [which runs] in the spinal nerves to the spinal cord.[3]

We are continually tending to lose our balance, slipping, sliding, falling—and recovering. Some of the muscles are particularly well placed to be stretched and pulled by every movement of the body: these are the muscles in the neck which hold the skull firmly on top of the spine. They are very well supplied with spindles. When the head moves on the neck some of these muscles are bound to be stretched and the spindles stimulated. The excitation is then transmitted in the usual way to the [spinal] cord. But within the cord these impulses are relayed not only to the lower motor neurons at the same level which will convey them to the neck muscles, but also to muscles lying in many other parts of the body: the effect is to cause such contraction as is necessary to bring the body back again to the upright position. These neck reflexes are very important indeed in helping us to regain our balance.[4]

You will never feel a spindle in action while you study the Alexander Technique. But you will think, react, and behave differently once you become aware of your Primary Control. 'How it works' is in the end unrelated to 'how *you* make *it* work'. This applies universally. A physiological understanding of the vocal organ, for instance, will not necessarily help you sing better.

3. *Positioning the head.* To use the Primary Control well does not mean to hold your head in the right position. Alexander speaks of a *relativity* of the head to the neck, and of these to the back. This implies a dynamic balance, an ever-changing relationship in which fixity has no place. As you walk, sit, stand, speak, or play the violin, you adjust your Primary Control constantly. Further, your active understanding of the Primary Control will change as you learn and grow. Therefore the relationship of head, neck, and back is fluid both in the short and in the long term. And so it should be. The photographs of Pablo Casals (Fig. 2), Janos Starker (Fig. 3), Art Blakey (Fig. 4), and Jascha Heifetz (Fig. 5) illustrate that there is no 'right position' for the head. Casals's head drops forwards slightly, Blakey's backwards; the heads of both Starker and Heifetz are straight. Yet all four men use their Primary Control well. The spine is neither contracted nor slack.

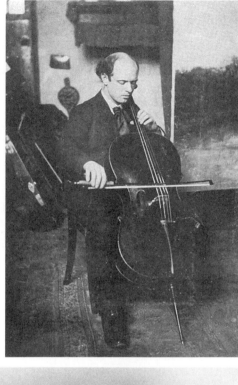

FIG. 2 (right). Pablo Casals

FIG. 3 (below). Janos Starker

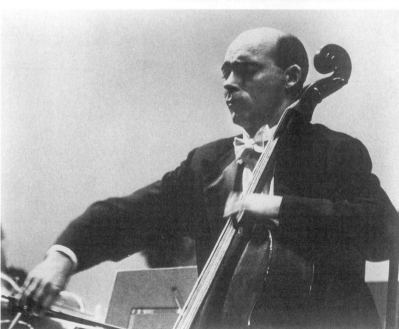

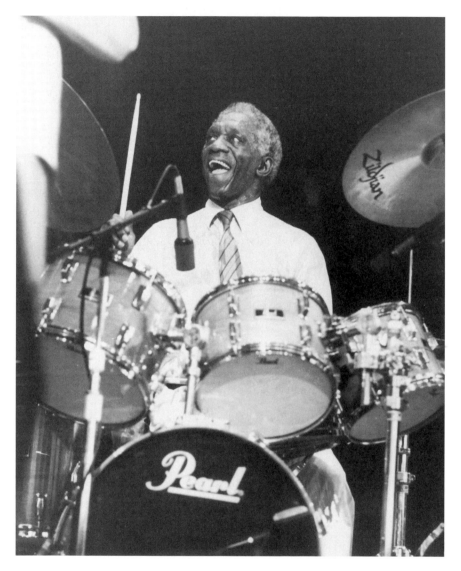

FIG. 4. Art Blakey at Ronnie Scott's in London

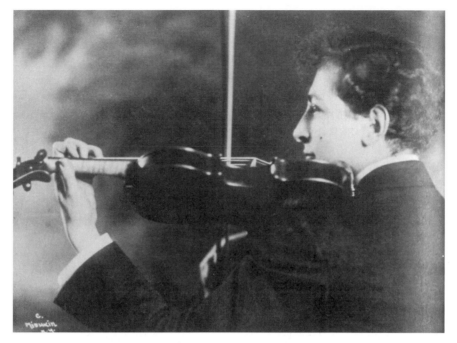

FIG. 5. The young Jascha Heifetz

The back is lengthening and widening, the shoulders are broadening. The neck remains an extension of the spine, allowing the head to move freely on the joint between skull and neck. Their entire bodies are oriented upwards, and their energies outwards.

4. *Non-doing*. To use the Primary Control well does not entail your doing the right thing. Rather, it requires that you stop doing the wrong thing. This does not involve the same type of muscular acts needed for you to lift an object or open a door. There are no physical exercises to improve the Primary Control. Instead, you must first stop contracting your head into your neck, and then prevent this contraction from recurring. I shall discuss the *cessation* and *inhibition* of unneeded activity in Chapter 4.

Changing the Primary Control

There are many ways of changing the use of the Primary Control. In the case of the cellist who twists his head around to look at his left hand, I have the following choices:

1. Have him play the cello blindfolded, in the dark, or with his eyes closed. This breaks up a habitual pattern of conception and misuse. At first Mark may become disoriented and lose whatever little control he normally has at the cello. But soon he will realize that he is quite able to play the cello without looking at his hand, and he will free himself from his familiar constraints.

2. Have him play the cello looking at me at the same time. As in the previous example, this makes it clear that looking at his hand is unjustified from a cellistic point of view. There would be no merit for Mark simply to fix his head in a new position. As Mark plays I may walk around the room, so that he has to turn his head from side to side to look at me. This decreases the likelihood of his positioning his head rigidly. If Mark feels uncomfortable looking at a listener (and he might, since he normally prefers to look at his own hands), I may ask him to look around the room, out of the window, or at himself in a mirror.

3. Have him play the cello while I manipulate his head and neck in the Alexander fashion, actively preventing him from misusing his Primary Control. This is extremely effective, provided that I use my hands well.

In many ways the hands-on approach is superior to all others. Misuse of the Primary Control is not determined solely by the use of the eyes. A violinist misuses his head, neck, and back as he tries to hold his violin up between chin and shoulder. A flautist twists her head, neck, and torso as she brings her flute to her mouth. A singer contracts her head into her spine even as she opens her mouth.

The hands-on approach of a well-trained Alexander teacher addresses all these different instances of misuse. Further, it ensures that what changes in the Primary Control is not the position of the head, but the relativity of head to neck and back. Finally, it ensures that the means of change is not something you do with the head and neck, but something that you stop doing—namely, contracting your head into your neck.

It is difficult, if not impossible, to describe accurately the quality of muscle tone an Alexander teacher seeks to obtain in her pupil's body. Good use of the Primary Control has nothing to do with the twisting of head and neck that you may do in the warm-up to dance classes, for instance. Neither does it involve the alternating tensing and relaxing that you learn in relaxation classes. Rather, it requires a combination of stretch of the spine and mobility of the head that is unlikely anything produced by habitual muscular doing. I shall address this issue again in Chapter 5, 'Direction'.

The improvement in Mark's Primary Control (guided by my hands or otherwise) has startling consequences. By changing the way he uses his head, neck, and back Mark affects his total co-ordination, and starts using his arms and hands differently as well. As a result there are noticeable improvements in his sound-production and in his use of his left hand. By *not* paying undue attention to the left hand, then, Mark becomes better able to control it. In general terms, the partial pattern (of left hand) becomes secondary and subservient to the total pattern (of head, neck, and back).

The Primary Control and Functioning

Let us consider Alexander's observations about the Primary Control and its relation to use and functioning:

I [cannot] enable my pupils to control the functioning of their organs, systems, or reflexes *directly*, but by teaching them to employ consciously the primary control of their use I [can] put them in command of the means whereby their functioning generally can be *indirectly* controlled.[5]

In cases where the knowledge of how to direct the primary control has led to a change for the better in the manner of the use of the mechanisms throughout the organism, the results of this 'conditioning' *can safely be left to take their own form.*[6]

In the previous chapter I wrote of habit as the manifestation of a constant. To eliminate a habit, change the conditions that allow the habit to exist. Make a change in the use of the self, and the habit (a manifestation of the use of the self) must necessarily change or disappear, even without your working on the habit itself. As Alexander says, the results of the basic changes in the use of the self can be left to take their own form. Condition the *total pattern*, and the *partial patterns* will look after themselves. 'The right employment of this primary control', wrote Alexander, '[leads] indirectly to the gradual disappearance of the defects; . . . indeed, these defects [are] found to be by-products of a wrong employment of the primary control.'[7]

This makes the Alexander Technique radically different from other methods of changing human behaviour. It seeks to alter use, not functioning; further, it seeks to alter use indirectly, through changes in the use of the Primary Control. You come to the Technique to 'cure' tendonitis or backache; by giving up the wish to remove the specific complaint and by working, instead, on improving the use of the whole self by improving the use of the Primary Control, you make positive changes in every sphere of your life, *and* you rid yourself of the specific complaint *in the process.*

We can now establish guidelines for solving all problems, be they 'physical', 'mental', 'technical', or 'musical'.

- Foremost in your mind when solving any problem should be to change the use of your Primary Control, or more precisely to *prevent interference* with its natural workings.
- At best, every procedure or exercise you pursue should *enhance* the natural workings of your Primary Control. Indeed, this should be the ultimate objective of every exercise.
- At worst, no procedure or exercise should ever *require that you misuse* your Primary Control. If an exercise does not enhance your Primary Control, it should at least not harm it. Do not be tempted by apparent benefits, short-term or otherwise, that may seem to accrue from an exercise if you know that you are misusing your Primary Control in executing it.

About Control

Alexander claimed that the 'how' of change in human behaviour is the theme of all his books. Talking of behaviour and of habit readily evokes the notion of control. Someone who recognizes the existence of an undesirable habit normally expresses a wish to control the habit, rather than being controlled by it. The very term 'Primary Control' would seem to indicate the possibility, and desirability, of control. This notion merits discussion.

There used to be a widely accepted image of human functioning. Man is like a car, his brain the driver. Today we think of the brain as a computer. These images both imply a driving, controlling force, and the ability of man to control himself as he would a machine. This is utterly false. As I mentioned earlier, in Alexander's view there is no distinction between the thing being controlled and the control itself. This precludes the possibility of mechanistic, manipulative control of human reaction. Alexander said that 'control should be in the process, not superimposed'.[8] This is a defining characteristic of the Technique, and a reason for its effectiveness.

Alexander's view of control has important practical applications. In an Alexander lesson, you will be tempted to improve your movements by controlling them. In all likelihood your movements will thereby acquire a rather unnatural, contrived quality—the contrary of what you should strive for. For your movements to become truly natural, you must give up whatever control you have of them. The very *idea* of controlling is a hindrance to changing your use. I shall discuss this issue further in Chapter 6, 'Action'.

'*I wish it to be understood*', wrote Alexander, '*that throughout [my writings] I use the term conscious guidance and control to indicate, primarily, a plane to be reached rather than a method of reaching it.*'[9] This idea has baffled many readers, but a passage by Cornelius L. Reid clarifies it:

A reasonable estimate of vocal potential can be made by observing the physical accomplishments of those who have achieved the highest levels of technical excellence. Among them are 1) an equalized tonal range extending over two and one-half octaves, 2) flexibility, 3) resonance and carrying power, 4) breath economy, 5) a sustained vocal line, 6) an even and unobtrusive vibrato, 7) durability, and 8) an ability to execute a *messa di voce* [a crescendo and decrescendo on a single long tone]. These attributes come with a built-in control system <u>which cannot be willed into being when vocal faults are present</u>.[10]

The great singer has great vocal control: he has reached a 'plane of conscious guidance and control'. But his control is the result of a voyage, not the means used to undertake the voyage itself. As implied in the passage above, to become a great singer think not of controlling your voice, but rather of eliminating vocal faults. The end result of the process of eliminating faults is control.

If control is a plane to be reached, not a method of reaching it, what exactly is this method of reaching control? We shall find the answer in examining human activity, and in seeing how we translate the thought of an action into action itself.

Think, Play, Judge

Let us choose a situation in which a specific act is desired: lifting an arm, saying a word, playing a musical phrase. Gerhard Mantel, in his book *Cello Technique*, refers to this as a 'goal-oriented movement'. He writes:

Any body movement is based on the following scheme:
1. We conceive a goal. This conception may be visually or acoustically determined, or it may be derived from our movement memory.
2. The brain sends motor impulses through the nerve pathways to the muscles. We need not go into the physiological details of those nerve pathways, except to say that each motor impulse consists of a series of pointlike single impulses. The frequency of the impulses and the number of muscle fibres involved determine the amplitude and the force of the movement, respectively.
3. A second system of nerve pathways reports success or failure to the brain, i.e., whether the goal was reached (feedback). In response the brain sends out correcting impulses. Their success or failure is also reported to the brain. We must imagine this circuit in uninterrupted activity.[11]

Frank Merrick, in *Practising the Piano*, describes the same chain of events and calls it 'Think, play, judge'.[12] Merrick credits this pithy formula to Theodor Leschetizky, the great Polish piano teacher whose pupils included Paderewski and Schnabel.

An Alternative

Most musicians would have no qualms about such a formula, which seems straightforward and indisputably 'true'. Alexander thought otherwise, however, revealing his genius yet again. He proposed the following scheme:

In the performance of any muscular action by conscious guidance and control there are four essential stages:
(1) The conception of the movement required;
(2) The inhibition of erroneous preconceived ideas which subconsciously suggest the manner in which the movement or series of movements should be performed;
(3) The new and conscious mental orders which will set in motion the muscular mechanism essential to the correct performance of the action;

(4) The movements (contractions and expansions) of the muscles which carry out the mental orders.[13]

Let us call this scheme 'conception, inhibition, direction, action'. (Alexander presupposed that feedback is constant, yet unreliable, as we shall see in the next chapter.) For a musician, this means 'think, get rid of wrong thoughts, think again, play'.

Contrasted with Mantel's scheme, Alexander's has two distinct features: inhibition and direction. If conscious guidance and control is a plane to be reached, inhibition and direction together comprise the method of reaching it. Before studying inhibition and direction, however, we must look at how we form conceptions in our minds.

3 Sensory Awareness and Conception

Faulty Sensory Awareness

I walk into the house of a stranger. At once I am struck by several smells: disinfectant, wood polish, cat litter. I meet the stranger. I smell cigarette smoke in his hair, alcohol and garlic in his breath, aftershave. The smells are strong and unmistakable. Yet the stranger cannot feel either the smells of his house or those he gives off himself. Alexander teachers refer to this phenomenon as *faulty sensory awareness*.

This example illustrates a faulty sense of smell, but all of our senses give us messages that we misinterpret or ignore. Most people, for instance, are surprised and displeased to hear how different their voices sound on a tape recording from how they imagine them to be. We see photographs of ourselves, and cannot believe our own eyes. Some musicians, even accomplished ones, cannot tell that they are playing or singing out of tune, or out of time.

Faulty sensory awareness is a nearly universal phenomenon. We can see it at work in people all around us. Yet, precisely because of our own faulty awareness, we think that we are immune from it! Pupils who start lessons in the Alexander Technique may come to a sudden realization of how wrong their sensations really are, and how badly they misuse themselves. Some pupils, rather than understanding that they are feeling their habitual misuses for the first time, believe that the Alexander Technique is the cause of their misuses, which seem new to them. This is one of the great traps of the Technique (as it is, indeed, of all music teaching): ignorance is bliss, and he that increases knowledge increases sorrow. To go beyond sorrow the teacher needs skill, and the pupil perseverance. Resourceful pupils will positively enjoy the discovery of their faulty sensory awareness. To feel new sensations, even of wrong things newly detected, is a source of pleasure.

Alexander used to say, 'Don't come to me unless, when I tell you you are wrong, you make up your mind to smile and be pleased.'[1] Experienced Alexandrians find the ability to admit being wrong extremely liberating.

In the beginning it is hard enough to accept that you may be wrong when you feel right. You may find it harder still, however, to accept that you may be right when you feel you are wrong. 'If your neck feels stiff,' Alexander would say, 'that is not to say your neck "is" stiff.'[2] You think that you are relaxed when you are tight; equally, you think that you are stiff when you are well co-ordinated. Sometimes after a lesson, a master-class, or a performance, you are convinced that you played horribly, only to hear your teacher or the public assure you that you played magnificently. (This is often the case when you 'let things happen' on stage.) Faulty sensory awareness is a double phenomenon, then: what is wrong feels right, and what is right feels wrong.

The instances of sensory delusion are numberless. I shall give more examples throughout the book; for the time being, let us accept that sensory awareness is faulty in most people, most of the time. Now let us consider the importance of this simple fact.

Opinions and Tastes

You play the viola in a string quartet. During a rehearsal the first violinist tells you that you play out of tune. You are quite sure that you play in tune; you think you are right and your colleague wrong. You then form an opinion of your colleague's musical competence and general character: he is wrong, you are right, and you do not much like him. This opinion, we note, has been shaped at least in part by a sensory impression—a feeling. 'We have to recognize', wrote Alexander, '. . . that our sensory peculiarities are the foundation of what we think of as our opinions, and that, in fact, nine out of ten of the opinions we form are rather the result of what we feel than what we think.'[3]

I give another example. Your viola teacher asks you not to raise your shoulders when you play forte; she points out that your sound becomes scratchy whenever you do so. Here you decide that your teacher is wrong on *two* counts. You are quite sure that you are not raising your shoulders; and your sound is, of course, beautiful.

Needless to say, you form an opinion of your teacher, much as you did of your colleague.

Here two observations emerge. You form your musical taste, in this illustration concerning the beauty of sound, in the same way that you form your opinions: through sensory awareness. As long as sensory awareness is faulty, taste risks being faulty too. Cornelius L. Reid writes that 'most expressions of taste in the form of "like" or "dislike" are bound to be prejudicial almost by definition'.[4] The old saying 'there is no disputing about tastes' merits re-evaluation: taste is debatable indeed. I shall further discuss taste later in this chapter, and in greater detail in Chapter 17, 'Aesthetic Judgements'.

Proprioception

Our second observation concerns sense itself. We all learn at school that we have five senses: sight, hearing, taste, touch, and smell. In truth, however, we have yet another sensory mechanism—not the 'sixth sense' that is popularly synonymous with intuition, but *proprioception*. Intuition is not equal in nature to the other senses; it is misleading to call it a sense at all. Proprioception, however, is a sense just like the other five, and should rightly be counted among them. But I fear the usage of the term 'sixth sense' for intuition is too well established for us to assign it to proprioception.

Dr Oliver Sacks writes:

We have five senses in which we glory and which we recognize and celebrate, senses that constitute the sensible world for us. But there are other senses—secret senses . . . —equally vital, but unrecognized, and unlauded. These senses, unconscious, automatic, had to be discovered. Historically, indeed, their discovery came late: what the Victorians vaguely called 'muscle sense'—the awareness of the relative position of trunk and limbs, derived from receptors in the joints and tendons, was only really defined (and named 'proprioception') in the 1890's.[5]

Let us go back to our last illustration. Your teacher tells you that you raise your shoulders when you play, something which you simply do not feel. Proprioception is that sense responsible for the gauging of the relative positions of your body and its parts. Your not feeling the positions of your shoulders is symptomatic of *faulty proprioception*.

Proprioception concerns itself with all aspects of muscular activity:

orientation in space, relative position of body parts, movement of body
and limbs, the gauging of effort and tension, the perception of fatigue,
static and dynamic balance. (The vestibular system in the inner ears
plays an important role in establishing and keeping balance, but it does
not bear sole responsibility for it. 'Proprioception, to a considerable
extent,' writes Dr Sacks, 'can compensate for defects in the inner ears.
Thus patients who have been surgically deprived of their labyrinths
. . . may learn to employ and to *enhance* their proprioception quite
wonderfully; in particular, to use the sensors in the vast latissimus dorsi
muscles of the back—the greatest, most mobile muscular expanse in
the body—as an accessory and novel balance organ, a pair of vast,
winglike proprioceptors.'[6])

For Alexandrians, proprioception is the most vital of all senses.
Musicians prize their hearing above all. Nevertheless, it is possible for
a musician to be virtually deaf and yet, thanks to proprioception, adept
at music-making: witness the remarkable case of the percussionist
Evelyn Glennie. It is impossible for a musician to make music, however, if he is void of proprioception. 'If proprioception is completely
knocked out,' writes Dr Sacks, 'the body becomes, so to speak, blind
and deaf to itself—and (as the meaning of the Latin root *proprius* hints)
ceases to "own" itself, to feel itself as itself.'[7]

Dr Sacks writes that proprioception is unconscious and automatic.
'For normal man, in normal situations, [proprioceptive reflexes] simply do not exist.'[8] Yet this is not to say that proprioception *should* be
unconscious, or that it cannot be made conscious. George Coghill
wrote that Alexander 'demonstrated the very important psychological
principle that the proprioceptive system can be brought under conscious control, and can be educated to carry to the motor centres the
stimulus which is responsible for the muscular activity which brings
about the manner of working (use) of the mechanism of correct
posture.'[9]

Alexander's genius consisted in (1) understanding that your conception of movement, of action, of yourself, of others—your conception
of life—is entirely dependent on sensory perception; (2) highlighting
the importance of proprioception in relation to the total use of the self;
(3) realizing the pervasiveness of faulty sensory awareness; and (4) developing a method for bringing proprioception into the sphere of conscious, reliable guidance and control. To see how we can re-educate
our sensory awareness and thereby make it reliable, it is useful to understand how it first becomes unreliable.

The Causes of Faulty Awareness

There are several distinct reasons for the malfunctioning of our senses. First, the mind has an innate tendency to seek out the stimulation of the new, which necessarily crowds out the old. 'The aspects of things that are most important for us are hidden because of their simplicity and familiarity,' wrote Wittgenstein. 'One is unable to notice something because it is always before one's eyes.'[10] Once we become used to something we are likely to stop noticing it. Often it is only when a certain sound stops—the humming of a refrigerator, for instance—that we realize that it was there all along. It is useful to think of background and foreground: we push the habitual and familiar to the mind's background, so that the new and unfamiliar can take its prominent place in the foreground. Thus I smell the odours of a stranger right away, and forget my own rather too easily.

Second, the senses may become debauched through over- or underuse. The stranger of my example may be unable to sniff out new odours. He drinks and smokes heavily, his nasal passages are blocked, his sinus congested, his taste buds over-stimulated by spicy foods.

Third, the senses may be inadequate at birth, or become so through illness or accident.

Fourth, and most important for the Alexander teacher, the senses may become unreliable through misuse of the self. To clarify the relation of use to perception, I should like to quote an experiment described by Gerhard Mantel.

Imagine that you are holding two ten-litre buckets, one of them empty, the other filled with nine-and-a-half litres of water. Add a half-litre of water to the first bucket. You can immediately gauge the difference in the bucket's weight, through the mechanisms of your neck, shoulders, arms, and back.

Now add a half-litre to the second bucket. You will find it difficult, if not impossible, to tell the difference between nine-and-a-half and ten litres of water. The tensed arm, or rather the tensed body, that holds a heavy bucket loses sensitivity to differences in weight after a certain weight has been reached.

The freer a body part is, the better able it is to sense accurately what it is doing. When you misuse yourself you over-contract some parts of the body, and leave others too slack. The whole self suffers, including head, neck, and back. Every time you contract your neck you disturb its many proprioceptors and distort their feedback. Misuse, in other words, always causes a distortion of sensory perception.

Conception and Experience

I preceded this chapter with a discussion of the chain of events that lead to the execution of every muscular action: conception, inhibition, direction, and action. To conceive is to think of what you want to do, and how you want to do it. (The 'what' and the 'how' are one and the same, as we shall see in the next chapter.)

Many different factors contribute to the shaping of conception, but the most important of these is experience. (Another is imitation, which merits a chapter apart.) For instance, my conception of the simple gesture of sitting down and standing up is shaped largely by the accumulated memory of the many times I have performed the gesture—that is, my experience of it.

What links experience to conception is sensory awareness. I play a phrase on the cello. I receive kinaesthetic and aural impressions from my own playing: the phrase feels and sounds a certain way to me. I may like it or dislike it; in either case I form a conception in my mind of how I wish to play this phrase. Next time around this conception will shape my playing. Thus *experience shapes conception, and conception shapes experience.*

Clearly there is a vicious circle at work here. You cannot perform an act correctly until you have had the experience of performing it, and you cannot have the experience without performing the act. This circle, kept closed by faulty sensory awareness, is one of the great stumbling-blocks of musical pedagogy. Every time a music teacher (or singing coach, or conductor) asks a pupil to do something, the pupil *interprets* the teacher's instructions according to his habitual, faulty sensory perception, *executes* the now-distorted instructions with his habitual misuse, and *judges* the results of his own playing through faulty sensory perception. Thus every step a musician takes in learning to play takes him ever further away from his desired ends, *as long as faulty sensory awareness conditions both his conceptions and his experiences.*

This process affects all activity. A dialogue, for instance—between teacher and pupil, amongst colleagues in an ensemble, between people in daily life—is often a distorted exchange of distorted views, causing, as it frequently does, disagreement, bad feelings, and sometimes even war. It would be eminently useful, then, to break free from faulty sensory awareness and the misconceptions it entails.

When you change your use, you go inevitably through new experiences and sensations. Being unfamiliar, these experiences may feel wrong—so wrong that you will not want to go through them, necessary as they may be. *'People don't do what they feel to be wrong when they are trying to be right,'* Alexander wrote.[11] He found that he could better guide or goad pupils to do what felt wrong to them by touching and manipulating them.

It is true that many music teachers resort to using their hands to help their pupils, but there are important differences between the touch of an Alexander teacher and that of a music teacher. An Alexander teacher has spent hundreds of hours refining the use of her hands. She may use her hands to give a pupil the experience of a specific act—for instance, a bow-stroke, or the holding of an oboe—just as a music teacher would. More important, however, she is primarily concerned with helping a pupil develop good use of the whole self on a general basis. Further, she is able to produce effects as needed, directly *or indirectly* (affecting a pupil's neck by working on his hips and legs, for instance), thereby avoiding any end-gaining in the process. By bringing inhibition to the fore, she makes sure that rather than *doing* the right thing the pupil *stops doing* the wrong thing. Lastly, by using directions she avoids the traps of body mechanics and of classical conditioning. I shall discuss inhibition and direction in the next two chapters.

The vicious circle of faulty experience and faulty conception is broken, then, in two ways. The Alexander teacher gives you a new experience, untainted by your preconceptions or by the memory of previous attempts. Further, the improvement in your use, brought about by new experience, causes an automatic, indirect improvement in your sensory awareness. On the one hand, you bypass your habitual ideas of right and wrong; on the other hand, you become better able to gauge right and wrong objectively.

Improving Sensory Awareness

It is often useless to tell a pupil that he is doing something wrong; he will not necessarily feel it by being told about it. It may be useless too to tell him to do the right thing, as he will probably be unwilling or unable to do something of which he has no conception.

The most productive way of working is to give the pupil an experience of good use that contrasts with what he normally does. There are two mechanisms at work here. First, a change of use for the better entails an automatic improvement in sensory perception (according to the buckets-of-water principle). Second, the new experience brings with it a wealth of new sensations, which the mind pounces upon at once (according to the background–foreground principle), awakening the pupil's capacity to compare and discern. In other words, do not tell a pupil that what he is doing is wrong; give him something new and different to do, and let him come himself to the realization that what he was doing before was indeed wrong.

The development of sensory awareness usually goes through three phases. At first you are able to feel things after they have happened. I put my hands on your shoulders and direct your awareness into what you are doing to them. My hands exert some expert pressure upon your shoulders; as a result you release them downwards and outwards. In retrospect you feel that you were indeed raising and contracting your shoulders.

Later on, I place my hands on your shoulders, which are now relaxed. As you turn your head from side to side, or play a chord at the piano, or lift a trumpet to your lips, you realize that you are beginning to contract your shoulders as before. In contrast with your previous response to my hands, now you feel things as they are happening—rather than retroactively.

Still later, I place my hands on your shoulders again. Before you play or sing, you become aware of a sneaking desire you have to lift your shoulders even as you prepare to move. You feel things before they happen—the first step in being able to inhibit misuse. Inhibition, indeed, is the cornerstone of the Alexander Technique, as we will see in the next chapter.

4 Inhibition

Misuse and its Motivating Force

Robert, a cellist, has a constricted, irregular left-hand vibrato. Anne, a pianist, wants to play with a bigger sound. But the harder she tries to play more loudly the stiffer she gets, and her sound becomes smaller and uglier. Kathryn, a singer, suffers from disabling stage fright. She is a talented and well-trained musician, and pleasing the audience is very important to her. But when she gets on stage she presents herself awkwardly, sings badly, and becomes thoroughly disheartened.

The problems experienced by these musicians have several points in common. An unruly vibrato, a small sound, and stage fright are all manifestations of general misuse. In Robert's case, for instance, it is not only the mechanisms of vibrato that suffer. His left-hand position changing is jerky, his left-hand articulation imprecise, his intonation unreliable. As he tries to concentrate on improving his problematic vibrato his bow-arm becomes unsteady. Further, his head is contracted into his neck and twisted sideways, his shoulders raised, his torso bent, his legs and feet contracted, his breathing constricted.

Vibrato, a partial pattern (as defined in our discussion of the Primary Control), is a function of the use of the self, a total pattern. So are sound-production and stage fright. To eliminate a faulty partial pattern it is necessary to co-ordinate the total pattern that activates and regulates the partial one.

Another characteristic of Robert's vibrato is that it is a *habitual and automatic reaction* to a certain stimulus. Every time Robert decides to vibrate, he triggers the misuse of the vibrato mechanism reflexly. Likewise, every time Anne decides to play loudly an automatic reaction takes place. And so with Kathryn.

Since Robert's very wish to vibrate sets an automatic misuse of the self, the only way he can change his vibrato is *to stop wanting to vibrate as he understands it*. Anne has to stop wanting to play loudly, and Kathryn must stop wanting to please her audience.

This is the central point of the Alexander Technique, and we call it *inhibition*. To inhibit is not to consent to a habitual reaction which causes a misuse, total or partial, of the self. Notice that the idea is not to inhibit misuse directly, but to aim to inhibit end-gaining, the motivation to act that causes the misuse. Therefore our cellist must inhibit not the wrong tensions in his left arm but the wish to vibrate, this wish being responsible for the onset of the tensions. Anne, the pianist, inhibits not the stiffening of her arms but her wish to play loudly. And Kathryn, the singer, inhibits not the symptoms of her stage fright but the desire to please her audience.

Yet, as Alexander wrote, 'the association of manner of use of the self and manner of reaction [on the one hand] and conditions of functioning [on the other hand] [is] so close that control of one depends upon control of the other'.[1] To inhibit interference with the Primary Control is very near, in character, to inhibiting the wishes, desires, and motivations that set up the interference in the first place. Even as Robert pays attention to preventing interferences to his Primary Control, he inhibits his desire to vibrate in his usual way.

An Illustration

Let us examine Robert's case in detail. The process of changing his vibrato can be taught in five distinct but interrelated phases.

1. The teacher first gives the pupil the verbal and manipulative instructions necessary to change his co-ordination on a general basis. This entails directing the head, neck, back, shoulders, arms, and legs.

2. The teacher then asks Robert to play a sustained note on the cello but *not to vibrate it* (Ex. 4.1). Many cellists find it difficult not to vibrate a note, so deeply ingrained is their habit of always trying to vibrate. Clearly the whole procedure depends, for its success, on the

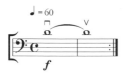

Ex. 4.1

willingness and ability of the pupil to inhibit his desire to vibrate and to stop his usual vibrato before he learns a new vibrato.

3. On a stringed instrument, the action of the right arm affects the action of the left arm, and vice versa. Let us call this interdependence the Bilateral Transfer. (I shall discuss this in Chapter 10, 'The Arms and Hands'.) Without an efficiently used bow-arm, the vibrato will invariably be faulty. While Robert inhibits any disturbances to his new and relatively improved use of the self, and while he inhibits his desire to vibrate, he must also seek to use his bow-arm with ease, in confident, firm, well-controlled motions that produce a sustained sound in forte dynamics. The better co-ordinated his bow-arm, the freer his vibrato will become.

4. The teacher can now place her left arm and hand over the pupil's left arm and hand, and gently but clearly initiate the rhythmic oscillations of the forearm that are the basis of a free, easily controlled, vocal-sounding vibrato. At this point, while the teacher moves the pupil's left arm, the pupil himself must continue to inhibit:

- any disturbances to his general co-ordination;
- his desire to vibrate; and
- any disruption to the continuity of gesture in his bow-arm.

The pupil must suspend temporarily his judgements of right and wrong, and not let his present musical taste interfere with his search for freedom. (I shall discuss this issue further in Chapter 17, 'Aesthetic Judgements.')

5. This experience may be made clear through repetition, variations in the verbal and manipulative instructions, and variations in the speed, amplitude, and direction of the vibrato. The teacher and pupil can experiment too with the very mechanism of vibrato. What makes vibrato 'right' is not a right mechanism, but a right way of using a mechanism, be it of the forearm, wrist, or hand.

Once the new experiences of vibrato become clearer, the teacher may ask the pupil to take over the responsibility for the activating of the vibrato. At first he does this intermittently: teacher and pupil take turns to activate the vibrato, attempting not to break the continuity of the gesture. Finally the teacher lets go entirely of the pupil's left arm, and allows the pupil to vibrate on his own.

This is only one of the many methods of working on vibrato. Cellists can improve their vibrato in connection with other functions of the left hand, such as articulation, pizzicato, and shifting. They can use certain mechanical exercises with the help of a metronome. They can rely on imitation, if the conditions are right. Nevertheless, inhibition should play a fundamental role in all these different learning processes.

In the case of a cellist's vibrato, it is possible for an Alexander teacher to give the pupil the new experiences of the desired partial pattern. In other cases, the teacher will not be able to give the pupil a direct, hands-on experience of a specific gesture. The voice, for instance, can be affected *indirectly* only, through changes in the total pattern. (Some singing teachers end-gain, and try to affect their pupils' voices by manipulating their throats.) Yet, whether the hands of the teacher affect a total or a partial pattern, inhibition of the end-gaining desires that triggers misuse remains the key to the entire process of change.

When Robert succeeds in inhibiting his habitual vibrato, he is likely to experience two striking sensations, both of which we must discuss at length. First, his new vibrato is so different from his familiar one that Robert feels that it is not a 'real' vibrato, but some other sensation, a different musical effect altogether. Second, he may well feel as if he is not vibrating at all—the vibrato seems to be *doing itself*.

Let us start with the first of these two sensations, of the vibrato as 'something unlike a vibrato'. This merits a detour.

The 'What' and the 'How'

In an Alexander lesson, the teacher asks the pupil to sit down. If he does so in his familiar manner, he will trigger his habitual misuse and contract his head into his spine, thrust his chest forwards and his bottom backwards, curve his back, raise his shoulders, stiffen his arms, and constrict his breathing. (Not for a second do we assume that the pupil is conscious of all this.)

To change his use and move without harming himself, the pupil must resist the temptation to sit down as he does usually. He must ignore the teacher's order to sit down, ignore his own desire to sit down, ignore the accumulated memory of all previous performances of the act of sitting down, ignore the very thought of the chair behind him.

Instead, he must pay close attention to the verbal and hands-on guidance that the teacher gives him. These instructions help the pupil change his whole co-ordination and achieve a balance between tension and relaxation. Mobility, stability, strength, and flexibility all come into play. The pupil becomes aware of each component part of his use and of their working as a whole. He becomes able to participate in an action and to observe his very participation. He *does* some things, he *allows* others to happen.

Once the teacher and the pupil have established, together, some of these constants of co-ordination (which can be done, however incipiently, quite quickly), the teacher asks the pupil to bend his knees while at the same time preventing any disarrangement to his new use. This mental command to bend his knees, together with the help of the teacher's hands, will take the pupil to a sitting position, without his having to give himself the old mental command to sit down.

For all purposes, 'sitting down' and 'bending the knees' are two different acts, associated with two different sets of sensations, and triggered by two different mental commands. One act is habitual, performed mostly without awareness, and characterized by the pattern of misuse described earlier. The other act is unfamiliar, performed with awareness and uncontrolled control, and characterized by the well-co-ordinated working of the whole organism. The second gesture is not an improvement on the first one: it is a change from it, which is the ultimate goal of the Alexander Technique. Thus Robert's new vibrato is not an improvement on his old one, but a new entity altogether: new thought, new action, new sensation.

Non-Doing

Robert's second unfamiliar sensation—the feeling that he is not actually vibrating, but that the vibrato is 'doing itself'—also helps us understand the nature of the Alexander Technique. It may be useful to consider inhibition briefly as a physiological process. As we saw in our discussion of the Primary Control, the brain projects messages through the nerve pathways to the various muscular mechanisms. Sir Charles Sherrington wrote: 'I may seem to stress the preoccupation of the brain with muscle. Can we stress too much that preoccupation when any path we trace in the brain leads directly or indirectly to muscle?'[2] Inhibition should be preparatory to the execution of each and every action—an *emptying of the pathways* of the unchecked, automatic flow of habitual messages.

Husler and Rodd-Marling wrote that 'it is entirely unphysiological to try and eradicate bad habits by cultivating better habits'.[3] Inhibition consists not in doing something new, but in not doing something old. And yet this clearing of pathways, this non-doing, is in itself activity. 'It has been remarked that Life's aim is an act, not a thought,' wrote Sherrington. 'Today the dictum must be modified to admit that, often, to refrain from an act is no less an act than to commit one, because inhibition is co-equally with excitation a nervous activity.'[4] The violinist Carlos M. Ramos Mejia writes of the well-known fact that muscles are arranged in pairs, and that 'every muscle that contracts produces a reflex contraction in its antagonistic pair. By preparation [i.e. inhibition] we understand the action of our will to produce a relaxing of the antagonistic muscle.'[5]

Inhibition, or *non-doing*, means not using wrong tensions (such as the contraction of an antagonistic muscle in a pair). The term 'non-doing' has created much confusion. The words of Patrick Macdonald are the clearest in this respect: 'It is alright to do, as long as you do the right thing'.[6] Non-doing does not mean that you are flabby or collapsed, or play possum. 'The cult of passivity and so-called relaxation is one of the most dangerous developments of our times,' wrote Macdonald. 'Essentially, it, too, may represent a camouflage pattern—the double wish not to see the dangers and challenges of life, and not to be seen.'[7] Our non-doing simply means not doing anything that is not right and desirable. Under ideal conditions—when inhibition precedes and accompanies every action—activity becomes free from excessive tension, thereby appearing effortless to the doer and to the observer. Such is the case of Robert's new vibrato: it feels so easy and unencumbered that Robert is tempted to say, 'I am doing nothing!'—when in fact he is doing a lot. 'Of course, non-doing is a kind of doing, but it is very subtle,' wrote Macdonald. 'The difference is that, in doing, you do it, whereas in non-doing, it does you. Those of you who have never had practical experience of the Alexander Technique will probably find this difficult to understand.'[8]

Inhibition and Timing

As Alexander saw it, inhibition should always be the first step in the sequence of events leading up to activity. There is a time element to inhibition. In the early stages of Alexandrian re-education, when inhibition is brought to the fore, it may well be necessary to wait some time after choosing a given act (sitting down, turning the head, playing a bow-stroke) and before actually proceeding with it, the better to prevent misuse. Alexander teachers often say that to inhibit is 'to stop and say "no".' In this sense inhibition is synonymous with waiting. Musicians have long appreciated the value of stopping and waiting. Singers, for instance, are familiar with the old saying, 'Think ten times and sing once.' (I discuss the applications of inhibition-as-waiting to music-making in Chapter 19, 'Delayed Continuity'.) We often do not realize how prevalent the habit of *not* waiting really is. Waiting—the temporary suspension of activity in daily life—makes social intercourse possible. Many conventions require it: stopping at a red light, for instance, or forming a queue at the checkout. There is great scope for its cultivation, be it in an Alexander context or otherwise. It is the backbone of good sense and of civility, two qualities dear to every committed Alexandrian.

Waiting is also an indispensable learning tool. Most music teachers have had the experience of teaching a pupil who will not stop his playing for long enough to listen to what the teacher has to say. The pupil carries on in his habitual manner, without having heard what the teacher said or having understood what she meant.

As a cello teacher I often resort to removing the bow and the cello from the hands of an over-eager pupil while I give some suggestion or advice, and I will not return his instrument until I am fairly certain that he has taken in the information offered. He does not wait because *he wants to be right.* Sooner or later the pupil understands the nature of his behaviour. Waiting eventually becomes symptomatic of his *giving up the eagerness to be right.* It is then synonymous with inhibition.

Inhibition-as-waiting is keenly needed, too, in situations where the activity taking place is eminently intellectual. Take the example of ear-training. I play a simple four-bar melody four times. I ask you not to try to write it down the first time around, but simply to listen to it. The second time I play it, I ask you to establish the key of the melody and write down its rhythm. The third time around I ask you to discern melodic patterns and underlying harmonies, and the fourth time around I ask you to write down the complete melody. This is a logical step-by-step procedure that should be easy to follow. Yet in most ear-training classes there always are students who panic and feel utterly incapable of taking down dictation. Rather than follow my simple instructions, they so worry about the *last* step of the exercise that they neglect the means whereby this step may be accomplished. They end-gain and try to write down the complete melody after the first playing of it. The solution to their woes is to inhibit: to wait before responding, and to stop wishing to get it right.

Timing, then, is an element of inhibition, but it does not define it. 'When you are asked not to do something,' Alexander said, 'instead of making the decision not to do it, you try to prevent yourself from doing it. But this only means that you decide to do it, and then use muscle tension to prevent yourself from doing it.'[9] Inhibition is not simply the temporary suspension of an activity: it is the suspension of the very wish to act. Mark Twain was fond of berating people who try to stop drinking, when what they really need is to stop wanting to drink.

Continuity of Inhibition

The issue of timing in inhibition deserves further consideration. To say that inhibition precedes every action is not to say that it stops once the action takes place. Robert must inhibit his desire to vibrate in his habitual way before he starts to play, and *continue to inhibit it* even as he plays and uses his newly found mechanisms of the left arm. Indeed, inhibition is continuous. Further, since the stimulation of life itself is continuous, there is a never-ending supply of habitual reactions to be inhibited anew. For instance, I inhibit my tendency to press too hard with my bow as I start a note on the cello; immediately afterwards I inhibit my tendency to draw my bow too quickly; immediately afterwards I inhibit my tendency to let the bow skate on the string as I finish my stroke. And so on, *ad infinitum*.

Inhibition never stops. Indeed, all human beings are inhibiting at all times; average people do not inhibit well, but that is not to say they do not inhibit at all. It is useful to recall Sherrington's words and consider inhibition as the neurological opposite of excitation. The organism is always in a state of mixed inhibition and excitation. For instance, when Robert vibrates at the cello he inhibits certain mechanisms of the neck, shoulders, and arms and excites certain other mechanisms, including those of the back and legs.

We could perhaps call *volition* the ability to inhibit and excite the self as each situation demands. The Alexander Technique makes conscious, selective, and effective what takes place unconsciously and more or less haphazardly in daily life. In Alexander's words:

The wild cat stalking its quarry inhibits the desire to spring prematurely, and controls to a deliberate end its eagerness for the instant gratification of a natural appetite. . . . In animals the inherited power [to inhibit] is there; in man also the power is there as a matter of physical inheritance, but with what added possibilities due to the accumulated experience gained from the conscious use of this wonderful force.[10]

When first bringing inhibition to the realm of consciousness, you may well need to exaggerate its waiting component, the temporary suspension of activity. But experienced Alexander pupils can and should inhibit *in motion*, without undue fear or hesitation. A flash of habitual thought is enough to set in motion habitual misuse. (If I attach electrodes to your buttocks and say the word 'chair', the electrodes will register a significant response regardless of how passive you pretend to be.) Given the right conditions, a flash of a different thought—co-ordinative, integrative thought—will set in motion co-ordinated, integrated activity. You need not and should not confuse hesitation with inhibition.

Inhibition unlocks the entire process of self-discovery that we call the Alexander Technique. It makes the Technique a far-reaching method of change, since it affects every facet of an individual's life. It also makes the Technique difficult to learn. As Alexander wrote, to inhibit is to delay the instant gratification of a desire. In this sense inhibition is a form of self-denial: when you inhibit, you deny yourself your wish to react in your habitual manner. Most people find this a struggle, despite the immense rewards inhibition offers. Further, Alexandrian non-doing goes right against our long-established wish to get results by *doing* something, and by being seen to be doing something.

Remember Alexander's words: 'Talk about a man's individuality and character: it's the way he uses himself.' To change your use you must necessarily give up your individuality *as you see it today*, and you are likely to put up a good fight. What is right feels wrong, and what is wrong feels right. In Part III of this book I shall discuss various ways of applying inhibition to music-making, but the best place for a musician to start learning about inhibition is not at his instrument (where he has invested so much emotionally) but in the simple acts of daily life.

5 *Direction*

Thought in Action

I sight-read a string quartet with friends. As I look at the score I grasp the essentials of the piece's formal structure, which help me make decisions regarding smaller sections and phrases. I conceive certain sounds, articulations, and dynamics; I command my arms, hands, and fingers to move as needed to make these imagined sounds real.

As I play I listen to the violins and the viola, and I look up from the music constantly to communicate visually with the other players. I think of what I will offer my friends to drink in a few minutes. I also have remembered a terribly funny joke that I must tell the second violinist, but I inhibit both my desire to tell this joke and my urge to laugh. My bladder is full, but I inhibit my impulse to empty it. Throughout the rehearsal I think of my head, neck, and back.

Most musicians will find the above scenario in no way extraordinary: it exemplifies what usually happens in practice, rehearsal, or performance. For the purposes of our discussion this illustration is useful because it shows many different aspects of *thought in action*. The Alexandrian concept of 'direction' brings something of relevance to bear upon every one of these aspects.

Unity of the Self

In my imagined situation, every thought of mine manifests itself as a bodily reality. This is true of my understanding of the piece's structure, of my decisions regarding bowing and fingering, and of my desire to laugh. Similarly, everything I do with my body is the result of a command from my brain—drawing the bow, turning my head to look at the second violinist, or not emptying my bladder.

There is a constant connection between brain and muscle—between what I think and what I do. It is impossible to say of an act that it is purely 'mental' or purely 'physical'. To sight-read a score in my mind's ears may be a less intensely physical action than to carry my cello up four flights of stairs, but both are equally an act of my whole self.

In the Alexander Technique, to speak of 'directing' or 'sending directions' is to discuss thinking. But this does not mean isolated intellectual activity. To learn to direct is not 'to train the mind', or 'to train the body'. It is rather to establish, cultivate, and refine the connections between what you think and what you do.

Simultaneity

In my imagined situation, I think of and do many things at the same time. This is true of every situation in daily life. Sometimes I do but two or three things, at other times many more. But it never happens that I do one thing, and one thing only. The Alexander Technique develops your innate ability of attending to several things at once in a specific way, namely in thinking of your use at the same time that you carry out any tasks of daily life.

To direct and make music should not put you out; after all, you have long been able to think of many things at the same time. You may claim that you need to 'concentrate' on your playing, to the exclusion of all other thoughts. Directing your use means simply paying attention to the means you need to achieve an end. To say that paying attention to the means would make it harder to achieve the end is a patent absurdity. I shall discuss concentration presently.

To Do, not to Do, to Stop Doing

In my imagined situation, some of the commands I give myself are for me *to do* something: draw a bow, turn a page, look at the violist. Other commands are for me *not to do* something: not to tighten my left arm when I change positions, not to hunch my shoulders for string crossings, not to laugh at a remembered joke. Other commands still are for me *to stop doing* something: to stop pressing my finger down into the string at the end of a note, to stop drawing my bow at the end of a phrase.

Some commands excite action, others inhibit it. At the cello or away from it, I am *always* in a state of combined excitation and inhibition. This is true for everybody all the time, regardless of how they use themselves.

Learning to direct allows you to change this balance of inhibition and excitation at will, thereby increasing your self-awareness and bettering your use. The most prevalent cause of misuse and poor functioning is a lack of inhibitory directions. Orders not to do and to stop doing should normally take precedence over directions to do.

Hierarchy

In my imagined situation, my understanding of musical structure and my ability to choose and execute bowings and fingerings are more important than my thinking of a joke, or of what to offer my friends to drink at the break. That there is a hierarchy of thought is indisputable. The Alexander Technique departs from accepted wisdom, however, in claiming that inhibiting the misuse of the Primary Control—the relationship between head, neck, and back—should be your most important thought in everything you do.

When I inhibit the interferences with the Primary Control I prevent a general pattern of misuse, since the Primary Control sets up the co-ordination of the whole self. Every aspect of my use and functioning—my sound, my rhythm, my ability to play and listen to my colleagues at the same time—improves when I inhibit a total pattern of misuse. By inhibiting a total pattern, I become better able to inhibit *or to excite* a partial pattern as well.

Let us call a total pattern of misuse 'pulling down', and a total pattern of good use 'thinking up'. If I inhibit my pulling down I am better able to inhibit my fear of high notes or my fear of fast bow-strokes. In effect these fears are but *manifestations* of my pulling down. When I think up, either I do not miss any high notes or, if I do, I am not unduly bothered and can carry on playing without missing the continuity of the musical line, which is more important than getting all the right notes. I inhibit my fears and, by carrying on despite failing here and there, I inhibit the frustrations that would otherwise feed my fears. The directions that prevent the misuse of the Primary Control are called *primary directions*, and I shall describe them later.

Awareness and Automatism

In my imagined situation, I am fully aware of some of the commands that I give myself; of some others I am only partially aware, or even not aware at all. In principle, this is just as well: a measure of automatism is an integral part of good co-ordination. Yet some of my automatic

commands hinder my playing, rather than help it. Alexandrian directing addresses the double problem of awareness and efficiency. By becoming conscious of commands you have always given automatically,
you learn to discern between useful commands and harmful ones. With
time you rid yourself of unnecessary directives from your brain, and
of the superfluous actions they entail. Further, the automatism of
Alexandrian commands is different in nature from that of commands
learned haphazardly. A habit acquired with good direction remains
accessible to the control of the will, so that it can always be re-exam-
ined, altered, or even discarded. (This type of automatism requires a
specific learning process, which I shall describe later in this chapter.)

Sooner or later, Alexandrian directing becomes efficient and automatic. When you first learn to direct, however, you may well feel
overly conscious of your every move, and you may also lose some of
the efficiency you had prior to studying the Alexander Technique. In
other words, things get worse before they get better. This is inevitable.
I mentioned it earlier in Chapter 3, 'Sensory Awareness and Conception', and I shall discuss it further in Chapter 17, 'Aesthetic Judgements'.

So far I have talked about ways in which Alexander directing is similar to ordinary thinking. In both there is a total union of body and
mind; in both there are concomitance and hierarchy of thoughts; in
both there are inhibitory and excitatory commands; in both there are
degrees of awareness and automatism. Directing might be better than
ordinary thinking in every one of these counts, but it does not *differ*
from ordinary thinking in any of them. Before going on with the practicalities of directing, however, it remains for us to see in what ways
directing is truly different from ordinary thinking.

A New Type of Direction

In describing my hypothetical sight-reading session, I mentioned that 'I think of my head, neck, and back'. This is quite vague;
let me be more precise. I think up along the spine, I direct my neck to
stay free, so that my head stays poised lightly on top of the spine, and
I direct my back upwards and outwards, so that it lengthens and widens. These directions differ in their nature from all the other thoughts
I have described so far, in that they do not result in any ordinary activity. They are not directions for me to do, or not to do, or to stop

doing something. 'Think up', 'let the neck be free', and so on are commands that I give myself without making an attempt to carry them out muscularly. To clarify matters, I should like to explain how, and why, one learns to direct in this manner.

In an Alexander lesson, I ask a pupil to think up along the spine. His first reaction will be to stiffen his neck, pull his head back and down, push his shoulders upwards and inwards, look up at the ceiling, hollow his back, and stop breathing, thereby assuming a posture that is but a caricature of a soldier in the marching line, or of a bad dancer. His reaction to my command is evidently undesirable. But all he did was to react to a new and unfamiliar stimulus in his old and familiar way.

I now ask my pupil to give up his first reaction. I place my hands on his head and neck and tell him not to do anything muscularly, but to let me gently stretch his spine. If I do my job well, I will take my pupil up along the spine. Let it be clear that the expression 'to think up' or 'to take somebody up' is shorthand for a total experience involving not only the spine but the head, neck, back, legs, and entire body, and having immediate psychological and emotional resonances.

To think up does not mean actively to lengthen the spine. Rather, it means to stop contracting it, and to let it return to its optimal length. My hands help the pupil understand what it is like to let the spine lengthen. In time the pupil translates the direction 'to think up' not as a muscular activity, but as an energizing which precedes and accompanies ordinary muscular activity—a direction not to *do the right thing*, but to *stop doing the wrong thing*.

There are many other such directions: point your shoulders sideways and apart; point your elbows out, away from your shoulders and away from one another; point your knees apart, away from the hips and away from one another; point your heels down; and others still.

Directing and Other Activities of Mind

To direct is always to think, but to think is not always to direct. It may be useful to consider how directing differs from types of thinking that are *not* directing.

In directing there is a quality of insistent, repeated thought. Alexander pupils have at times confused this quality with that of positive thinking, meditation, visualization, and self-hypnosis. To direct means to link a mental command, a tangible physical reality, and a sensorial feedback. In positive thinking and in visualization, this triple linkage is absent. My head is not a balloon; to imagine it so does not correspond to a tangent physical reality, but to command my head to go forwards and up does. The aim of meditation and self-hypnosis is a slowing down of the conscious mind; the aim of directing is a *quickening* of it.

This is not to say that visualization, meditation, and so on are useless or inherently negative. Learn how to direct first, and then bring your knowledge of how to link a thought, its resulting action, and its accompanying feedback to bear on all other activities of the mind.

If I am fully responsive to an image, I can use it to cause a healthy imitative reaction. I watch Fred Astaire dancing, Artur Rubinstein playing the piano, or Steve Cram setting his mile record, and I am inspired to embody what I observe. But if I use myself badly and suffer from faulty sensory awareness, to visualize setting a mile record will only disco-ordinate me further. 'There was a crooked man who ran a crooked mile.' When the crooked man visualizes, he translates an image into a distorted gesture.

Directing and Words

For the badly co-ordinated adult who learns good use almost from scratch, directing only becomes natural after a painstaking process which includes abstraction, analogy, and the use of words as aids to directing. In an Alexander lesson the teacher uses her hands at the same time that she verbalizes various directions. In time the pupil comes to associate the experiences and sensations of directing with their respective verbal commands. He can then use words to recall experiences, or even to trigger them. The words become a mnemonic index of sorts: 'thinking up' means a certain experience, 'heels down, knees apart' another, 'shoulders sideways and apart' yet another.

This is not to say that the Alexander Technique is akin to classical conditioning. The quickening of the conscious mind brought about by directing and required of it ensures that your reactions remain *choices* rather than automatic reflexes. When you say, in your mind, 'Think up', you remind yourself of your choices—to think up or not. The words do not trigger a set reaction. In fact you can use them to *break down* automatic reaction, rather than to arouse it, as I discuss presently.

There is a certain syntax to directing. If I say, 'Let the head go forward and up,' three distinct elements interact in a precise way. There is the action: to let it go; there is the part acted upon: the head; there is the orientation in space: forward and up.

Different parts of the self require different actions and orientations in space. I will not set down all the possible combinations, as I do not wish to give the reader the impression that he can learn to direct from a table of words. I give a few examples, with a view to illustrate certain points about directions.

- Actions: to let, to allow, to point, to push, to release, to tighten, to think, and so on.
- Body parts: the head, neck, spine, back, shoulders, arms, wrists, hands, fingers, legs, knees, heels, toes, lips, tongue, jaw, and so on.
- Orientation in space: up, down, in, out, backwards, forwards, sideways, apart, and so on. This could also be a muscular state: free, long, broad, firm, and so on.

To illustrate the use of words in directing, let us consider the directions for the Primary Control: Let the neck be free, to let the head go forward and up, to let the back lengthen and widen, *all together, one after the other.*

'Forward and up' is undoubtedly the more confusing of these directions; it has often been understood as a position of the head, which it most emphatically is not. Alexander threw his hands up in the air when he tried to explain it, and claimed that you needed to be given the experience to understand it. Patrick Macdonald stated, rather more helpfully, that

it is useful to consider the 'forward' as an unlocking of the head at the atlanto-occipital joint [between the skull and the spine] by refraining from tightening and pulling it backwards in the accustomed way, and the 'up' as a tiny extension of the spine, which is achieved following this unlocking. The movement, if any, is, in an experienced pupil, so small as to be hardly a movement at all. It is a directed flow of force or a kind of pulsation, no more than a heart beat.[1]

Macdonald went on to explain the difference between a position and a direction. It is possible, although difficult, to direct the head forward and up even if it is going back and down in space. This is best illustrated by the picture of George Balanchine and Arthur Mitchell (Fig. 6).

Their positions in space are similar, but their directions quite different. Balanchine's head is directed forward and up, Mitchell's back and down.

About the all-important idea of sending various directions *'all together, one after the other'*, Alexander wrote that

> to maintain the unity that is involved in this connected series of acts, [the pupil] will have to continue to project the directions necessary to the performance of the first act of the series *concurrently* with projecting the directions necessary to the performance of the second, and so on throughout the series until all the preliminary acts have been performed in their connected sequence. . . . This process is analogous to the firing of a machine-gun from an aeroplane, where the machinery is so co-ordinated that each individual shot of the series is timed to pass between the blades of a propeller making 1,500 or more revolutions to the minute.[2]

When directing, you can use words in several ways. Ask yourself questions: 'Am I thinking up? Is my neck free? Am I taking my head forward and up?' Declare, in the first, second, or third person: 'I am thinking up and pointing my shoulders sideways and apart.' Exhort: 'Forward and up! Forward and up!' Caution: 'Don't pull down, don't contract, don't rush.' Run a list: 'Head, neck, back, spine, legs, knees, heels.' Use variety, imagination, and humour. Do not forget that the words are an aid to organizing the kinaesthetic experiences and not the experiences themselves. And keep in mind that sensorial experiences are nearly impossible to describe, but a little easier to demonstrate in a lesson.

Alexander did not always define his terms clearly. He came close to giving a precise definition of direction when he wrote: 'When I employ the words "direction" and "directed" with "use" in such phrases as "direction of my use" and "I directed the use," etc. I wish to indicate the process involved in projecting messages from the brain to the mechanisms and in conducting the energy necessary to the use of these mechanisms.'[3] In other words, directions are messages from the brain to the muscles via the nerves. These messages energize the self in various ways, according to need. I remind my readers of Gerhard Mantel's words: 'Each motor impulse [i.e. direction] consists of a series of pointlike single impulses. The frequency of the impulses and the number of muscle fibres involved determine the amplitude and the force of the movement, respectively.'[4]

Directions are a *process* involving the linking up of thought to action. One of the *results* of this process is the energizing of the body.

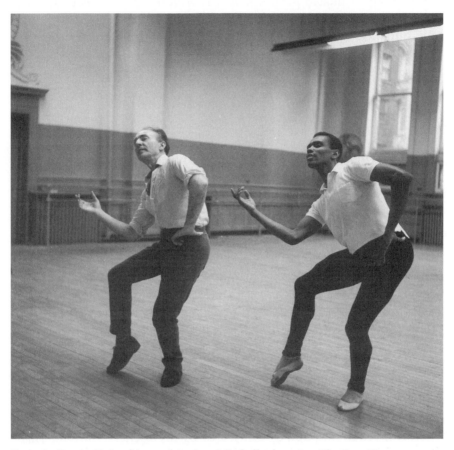

FIG. 6. George Balanchine and Arthur Mitchell rehearsing *The Four Temperaments* (1958)

When directing is healthy, it results in a particular muscular quality that is alive, elastic, vital. Sometimes Alexander teachers refer to the process by speaking of the result; they say of the elastic muscle tone of a well-co-ordinated person that it is *well directed*. This carries the risk of believing that the energies resulting from directing can be somehow obtained without reference to the thinking that creates them—a belief better avoided.

The Unity of the Self Reiterated

I write often of the utter impossibility of separating mind and body. Yet some of my words may well give the impression that directing is no more than simple body mechanics. Far from it. To direct is not to manipulate or control the body. It is an act of imagination and creativity, an act that brings together thought, sensation, movement, knowledge, perception, awareness. To direct is *to will*—to intend, to choose, to decide.

Further, my discussion so far covers but one aspect of directing. I tell a pupil to think up along the spine, to point his head forward and up and his back back and up, and to send his knees forward and away. These are 'directions to the parts'. But I also tell him to 'get out of the way', to trust my hands, to lose his balance, to move without fear or hesitation, to carry on watching, listening, and breathing. These are 'directions to the whole'. It is futile to insist on localized directions if the general attitude of my pupil prevents him from integrating his directions into a harmonious whole. Therefore, directive instructions— whether given to the pupil by himself or by his teacher—must alternate between those focused on specific parts of the body and those aimed at the whole. I shall discuss this point further in 'Concentration and Attention' at the end of this chapter.

Contraction and Expansion

Some readers may be surprised to find, in my list of possible directions, the word 'tighten'. If the aim of directing is freedom, should we not always avoid tightening? In reality good use of the self entails not boundless expansion but a perfect balance between expansion and contraction, which may be achieved only with the proper tensing of the body parts that *need* tensing.

A slack spine is almost never desirable: 'spinelessness', both literal and metaphorical, is anathema to the enlightened Alexandrian. When countering a slack spine, the direction 'tighten the spine' is wholly positive, provided that you translate it correctly. Other parts of the body may need tensing. A double-jointed pianist, for instance, may well have to learn to tighten some of his joints in order to have the necessary strength and stability in his playing fingers.

Anatomy, Physiology, and Directing

My list of body parts to be directed does not mention specific muscles or sets of muscles. Direct control of single muscles plays no part in acquiring good use. By commanding my arm to raise I cause the latissimus dorsi to work, but I cannot command the latissimus dorsi to work in order to raise my arms. Tobias Matthay, a piano teacher and writer who was Alexander's contemporary, wrote that

the attempted realization of the precise locality of the muscles concerned [in piano playing] is not only futile, but is bound to impede the learner's progress, since it must take his attention away from the points where it is most directly needed. . . . What we *can* learn and *should* teach is what may be termed the general *Muscular Mechanics* of the limbs we use. We can learn which section of the playing limb should be exerted and which should be left lax; and by thus willing the desirable LIMB-stresses into action and by inhibiting the undesirable ones, the concerned complex muscular co-ordinations will indirectly but surely be called into responsive action.[5]

Men and women whose co-ordination is naturally good often have little or no anatomical or physiological insight. To pass from bad to good use does not require this insight either, as witnessed by the successes of music teachers who rely not on mechanistic control but on the imagination of their pupils and their ability to *react differently with their whole beings* in a given situation—the ultimate purpose of directing. Knowledge of anatomy and physiology, although not strictly necessary, *may* be useful, but only if it does not tempt a pupil away from this purpose.

Tendencies and Oppositions

I wrote earlier that the Alexander Technique does not concern itself with bodily positions. I can now say that it concerns itself rather with the directions that exist within each position. Any position, held for however long or short a time, is 'right' if the interplay of directions within that position is right, and 'wrong' if otherwise.

This is a point easily demonstrated, but not so easily explained. It may be useful to think of directions as *tendencies*. Patrick Macdonald presents a pertinent analogy:

Consider a piece of steel in proximity to a magnet. We are told that even though the piece of steel does not move in space towards the magnet, every particle of the steel will be orientated towards it. Also, while keeping the orientation of the particles towards the magnet it is possible to move both magnet and steel in any direction, including the opposite direction in which the particles are orientated; the particles can be said to be pointing two ways at once.[6]

Similarly, you can move your body forwards in space while directing (or pointing) it backwards in the opposite direction. The body then *tends* backwards, even as you move it forwards. At rest, too, your body may tend upwards or downwards, forwards or backwards, and so on. 'Position, muscular movement, and "direction" are three different activities,' writes Macdonald; 'the third activity—"direction"—should go on inside the other two activities.'[7]

The ability of the body to move in one direction while tending towards another direction is essential to its well-being. Let us call this phenomenon 'opposition'. There are two types of opposition: between two or more parts within the self, and between the self and an exterior force bearing upon it. If I point my head forward and up and my back back and up, I set up an opposition between head and back; if I point my elbow out, away from my shoulder and from the trunk, and my wrist in, away from the elbow and towards my trunk, I set up an opposition between elbow and wrist. If you place your hand on my back and push me forwards, I point my back backwards against your touch and create an opposition between the two of us.

Opposition allows bodily positions to be stable and dynamic, and movement to be fluid and efficient. There are innumerable possibilities for opposition within and without the self. You need not consider the word 'opposition' negatively. When you dance with a partner—the waltz, the swing—it is the opposition (or resistance) between the two of you that allows you to move as one. I have already quoted G. B. Lamperti in my discussion of tension and relaxation:

Singing is accomplished by opposing motions and the measured balance between them.
   This causes the delusive appearance of rest and fixity—even of relaxation.[8]

The singing voice in reality is born of the clash of opposing principles, the tension of conflicting forces, brought to an equilibrium.[9]

Opposition can be extremely pleasurable in all its manifestations, be it dancing, blowing air through the reed of an oboe, drawing a bow across a string, or simply directing your head in opposition to your back.

Directing and the Breaking Down of Automatic Reactions

I claimed earlier that the Alexander Technique is not akin to classical conditioning—an extremely important point that merits a detour. Early on in his acting career Alexander started suffering from vocal problems. It was in examining and solving these problems that Alexander came to develop the technique that now bears his name. He told his story in full in the first chapter of *The Use of the Self*, which is required reading for all serious Alexander pupils. For the moment we are going to examine a single aspect of his fruitful journey.

Alexander determined that his vocal troubles were caused by the way he misused his whole self. He found, among other things, that he contracted his head into his neck every time he spoke or recited. It was obvious to him that the solution lay in his speaking without misusing his head and neck. Despite all his efforts, however, he found that he could not *think up* and *speak* at the same time; whenever he spoke, he invariably and automatically contracted his head into his neck. After much struggle he struck upon an original and insightful solution to his vocal problems.

To stop misusing himself when he spoke, Alexander would make the decision to speak but then refuse to carry it out. He understood that the automatism of a reaction lies not in the action itself, but in the link between the decision to act and the resulting action. Rather than eliminating his misuse, he needed *not to respond* to the stimulus which preceded the misuse itself.

Alexander then developed an effective strategy to solve his vocal troubles. You can use the same strategy to break down all your undesirable, automatic reactions. He would first give himself the directions for the co-ordinated use of his whole self—in short, he would *think up*—and would then decide to speak. Rather than going ahead and speaking, as he had always done, Alexander would then do one of three things:

1. carry on thinking up and do nothing;
2. carry on thinking up and do something other than speaking (raise his hand, for instance); or
3. carry on thinking up and speak.

By alternating freely between the different responses, and by choosing to *not* speak frequently, Alexander found that *thinking up* became gradually more important than speaking itself, and he was finally able to think up *and* speak at the same time.

Alexander wrote that you must 'separate the order [you] are asked to give from the act or acts of which it [the order] is the forerunner'.[10] 'The whole principle of volition and inhibition are [*sic*] implicit in the recognition of this differentiation.'[11]

You should be able, for instance, to give yourself the command to lift your arm and *not lift it if you so decide*, or to listen to the command 'think up' and *do nothing*. As a method, this is the contrary of classical conditioning; if you were a dog, the bell would ring and you would not salivate. There is no better way of acquiring complete control of your reactions in every situation. You may wish to reread the above section in connection with Chapters 18–21, where I suggest ways of applying Alexander's strategy to music-making.

Concentration and Attention

I wrote earlier of the *simultaneity of directions*. We are always thinking of more than one thing at a time. This is natural and desirable. Yet sometimes the wrong types of thoughts, or the wrong hierarchy of thoughts, cause 'mind wandering', for which the usual remedy is 'concentration'. Let us define the latter. Patrick Macdonald wrote that 'the meaning of the word "concentration" has been debased. It used to mean to relate a set of surrounding factors to a central point. It now very often means to separate a point from its surroundings.'[12]

Concentration as practised today means not only separating factors but eliminating them as well. Yet the true meaning of co-ordination lies in harmoniously integrating however many factors any situation may require. To separate or eliminate factors is a problem, not a solution. I explain.

In an Alexander lesson you learn to add certain thoughts to all your activities. These thoughts (or directions) make you aware of the use of your self, and they allow you to change your use at will. You direct your head, neck, and back even as you sit, stand, walk, speak, practise the piano, or perform in front of an audience. You are therefore always thinking of at least two things at the same time: your own use, and the activity in which you are engaged. You think up and speak; think up and walk; think up and play.

Most beginners, however, find it difficult to think up *and* react at the same time. They say, 'I have to concentrate on the piano; thinking of my neck distracts me from playing my best.' Or, 'I must stop playing to think up; let me just concentrate on my spine for a while.'

Yet, surely the Alexander Technique would be useless if you had to separate it from the activities of daily life. To concentrate on playing to the exclusion of the primary directions or to concentrate on directing to the exclusion of moving are both 'daggers of the mind', in Alexander's words. He wrote:

The essence of the religious outlook is that religion should not be kept in a compartment by itself, but that it should be the ever-present guiding principle underlying the 'daily round,' the 'common task.' So also it is possible to apply this principle of life [Alexandrian direction] in the daily round of one's activities without involving a loss of attention in these activities.'[13]

'If you do anything to affect the processes,' Alexander said, 'you must do something that will affect the results of these processes.'[14] The better you use yourself, the better you will play the piano; to concentrate on playing to the detriment of your primary directions can only make your playing worse.

To concentrate on thinking up along the spine creates its own problems. 'If I don't concentrate,' pupils say, 'I won't be able to feel what is going on.' This is demonstrably false. Macdonald presents the following scenario:

Teacher, tapping pupil on shoulder: 'Did you feel that?' *Pupil*: 'Yes.' *Teacher*: 'Did you try to feel it?' *Pupil*: 'No.' *Teacher*: 'In the same way, when I co-ordinate you with my hands, you need not try to feel what I do. If you do try, you will only interfere with what you ought to be registering.'[15]

It is easy to tell when a pupil is concentrating: he gazes in space without blinking, constricts his breathing, and stops speaking or listening. We could also call this 'self-hypnosis'. These are clearly not the best conditions for co-ordinating yourself.

Directing requires a quickening of the conscious mind, which increases your awareness of yourself, of others, and of the environment around you. Bruce Lee, the great martial artist and teacher, wrote that 'classical concentration . . . focuses on one thing and excludes all others, and awareness . . . is total and excludes nothing.'[16] 'A concentrated mind is not an attentive mind but a mind that is in the state of awareness can concentrate.'[17]

The difference between concentration and awareness is perfectly, yet unwittingly, illustrated by this excerpt on the fabled abilities of two great conductors, Erich Kleiber and his son, Carlos:

Erich Kleiber would go for long walks with a score in his hand and his children walking in front, immerse himself completely in whatever work he was preparing, but at the same time remain aware of everything going on around him. Once, he stopped his perusal long enough to save Carlos from an accident, and then calmly returned to his score. (Carlos' own concentration is no less amazing: when he made his début at La Scala in the 1974–75 season with *Der Rosenkavalier*, he continued to conduct throughout the Fruli earthquake, which shook the place, racked the chandeliers and emptied the gallery. 'I didn't notice!,' he said later, when he was told what had happened after complaining that the orchestra had seemed restless!)[18]

The elder Kleiber was *aware* of everything; his awareness being all-inclusive, he could *concentrate* on his score while keeping track of all around him. The younger Kleiber, however, *concentrates* on his music-making and becomes *unaware* of the world around him. (I hasten to add that Carlos Kleiber is perhaps the finest, and most Alexander-like, of all conductors working today. I imagine that he is capable of perfect awareness, but slips into concentration from time to time!)

Elsewhere in the book—notably in the next chapter, 'Action', and in Chapter 17, 'Aesthetic Judgements'—I shall further the discussion of attitude of mind, the passage from concentrating to being aware, the difficulties of making directions intuitive yet reliable, and the differences between self-consciousness and self-awareness. For now I quote the teacher Nicholas Brockbank: 'The key to successfully applying the Technique to ordinary life must be not to look as though you are. This should lead, in time, to not looking as though you need to.'[19]

6 *Action*

Ends and Means

When discussing inhibition, we saw that a habitual gesture—sitting down, for instance—is activated by a certain thought and is accompanied by certain feelings. Let us call these thought A, gesture A, and feeling A. A different, inhabitual gesture accomplished in a directed, Alexander-like manner—energizing the body upwards in order to bend the knees and lower yourself in space—is activated by a completely different thought and is associated with completely different sensations: thought B, gesture B, feeling B.

The main difference between these two gestures is that A is based on the end-gaining principle, and B on the means-whereby principle. In A, all that matters is to sit down. In B, self-awareness, inhibition, and direction take precedence over the act of sitting down.

We saw in the previous chapter that Alexander, when searching for a solution to his vocal problems, found a stumbling-block in that critical moment when the giving of directions merged into 'doing'. However well he directed his preparations for an act, he lost his directions when he went ahead with the act itself.

To put it succinctly, act A is wrong but feels right, and act B is right but feels wrong. At the decisive moment of action, the doer chooses invariably to do what *feels* right to him, not what *is* right. The solution, logically, requires that he abandon his ideas of what is right, and embrace what feels wrong. 'Paradoxical as it may seem,' wrote Alexander, 'the pupil's only chance of success lies, not in "trying to be right," but, on the contrary, in "wanting to be wrong," wrong, that is, according to any standard of his own.'[1] I believe there are four separate but interrelated factors in passing from wrong to right, and in achieving truly free action: giving up trying, giving up judging, ridding yourself of hesitation and eagerness, and timing your actions precisely.

Giving up Trying

'If at first you don't succeed, try, try, try again,' said the Victorians. Patrick Macdonald re-stated this pithy saying in light of the Alexander Technique: 'When at first you don't succeed, never try again, at least not in the same way.'[2] People often feel that failure comes from not trying hard enough, and follow failure with a greater determination to succeed and a corresponding increase in their misuse. Alexander wrote that a pupil has

to learn by experience that *trying* to gain his end, *trying* to be right, is the surest way to failure in carrying out his newly made and reasoned decision. He must become convinced by his own experiences that what he feels is right is wrong, and that the idea involved in trying to do better at one time than another is merely a myth, a 'dagger of the mind.'[3]

'Will-power' exerted by a pupil whose use of himself [is] misdirected would be exerted in the wrong direction. . . . It is not the degree of 'willing' or 'trying,' but the way in which the energy is directed, that is going to make the 'willing' or 'trying' effective.[4]

'Try again, this time with less tension' is a directive we all hear and give freely. If the intention and the desire behind an unsuccessful gesture remain the same, the gesture itself will remain unsuccessful, regardless of the amount of tension involved. A better directive, then, is 'don't try again; do something else altogether'.

Giving up Judging

If you are really going to pay attention not to the end, but to the means whereby the end may be achieved, then you should be happy enough to act even if you do not attain your end. Take the example of a pianist who has to find a chord at one extreme of the keyboard, in the midst of a fast passage that does not allow him much time to prepare the needed leap of the hand. If he misuses his playing arm, he will almost surely miss the chord. The very wish to attain his end and strike the chord accurately, however, causes him to stiffen his arm. Therefore, he has to be willing to miss the chord, so to free his arm, so to find the chord! (I shall discuss this example, and related ones, in Chapter 21, 'The Trampoline'.) And yet, because it 'feels wrong' to miss the chord and to have a free arm, the pianist will stiffen his arm every time—and miss the chord all the same.

Alexander pointed out that, if you are really paying attention to the means and not the ends, then you must be willing to act *'irrespective of whether, during the progress of the activities concerned, the performance is correct or incorrect.'*[5] Suspend your judgement of right and wrong and act with indifference to the end result of your actions. This is not to say that there is no right and no wrong, and that you are free to do any old thing; simply, your *feelings* of right and wrong are inaccurate and need to be bypassed if you are to attain true objectivity. One of my favourite Alexander sayings is also one of his most Zen-like: 'You all want to know if you're right. When you get further on you will be right, but you won't know it and won't want to know if you're right. . . . I don't want you to care a damn if you're right or not. Directly you don't care if you're right or not, the impending obstacle is gone.'[6]

To liberate yourself from the constraints of inaccurate feelings of right and wrong means both not to anticipate the outcome of your actions and not to judge them afterwards. (Notice that both are inhibitory, non-doing attitudes.) Bruce Lee speaks of combat, but his words apply aptly to music-making and to the learning of new gestures in the Alexander Technique:

The perfect way is only difficult for those who pick and choose. Do not like, do not dislike; all will then be clear.[7]

The great mistake is to anticipate the outcome of the engagement; you ought not to be thinking of whether it ends in victory or in defeat. Let nature take its course, and your tools will strike at the right moment.[8]

Tito Gobbi, the great singer who was noted for his outstanding acting abilities, speaks of a singer missing a gesture on stage:

One word of warning, however, to anyone adding these refinements [gestures and smiles] to his or her presentations: if any of these moments is messed or bungled, never look back on it until the performance is over. The moment has gone and can never be recalled. To dwell on it will only increase a sense of confusion which can quickly lead to disaster. To let even part of your mind be preoccupied with what has happened is like tossing the stone which starts the avalanche.[9]

To worry about a mistake in performance and to castigate yourself for it even as you perform are clearly undesirable. In daily practice and during an Alexander lesson the same principle applies. It is true that outside public performance you can stop, repeat a gesture, and correct a mistake. Even then, however, if you linger on a gesture's 'wrongness' as you execute it you risk stilting the gesture and making it irredeemably wrong. Execute your every gesture with *élan* and authority, whether it *is* wrong or it *feels* wrong, and stand back from the gesture and consider it with detachment.

Hesitation and Eagerness

Action that is not ideal is often marked by hesitation or by eagerness. Hesitation and eagerness both are forms of end-gaining behaviour. In one there are timidity, insecurity, feeble gestures that fall short of the goal, a false kind of relaxation. In the other there are brusqueness, excess effort and tension, hurry, angular motions that overreach their goal. Hirohide Ogawa, Zen teacher and basketball coach, encapsulates these two opposites nicely: 'A violent shot can break the post or tear the net, but it will not score. Neither will you impress me with a timid throw that falls short. Rage and fear, two more stepping-stones into the whirlpool.'[10]

This is not to say that people either hurry *or* hesitate: it is possible to do both, at different times or even together. An Alexander lesson affords a great many opportunities for the pupil to become aware of hesitation and eagerness, the constant passing from one to the other, and the effects that both have on the use of the self.

Cornelius L. Reid points out the apparent contradiction between two truthful sayings: 'He who hesitates is lost' and 'Look before you leap.' I think they can be thought of as one: 'Look before you leap, and don't hesitate once you have decided to jump.'

To look before you jump means to inhibit and to direct. Neither, however, should make you afraid to react. This is one of the great traps of the Alexander Technique: badly taught or badly learned, it may turn you into what we call an Alexandroid—someone stiff and careful, overly conscious of his own misuse, and afraid to squeak lest he end-gains. Keep in mind that to be afraid of end-gaining is to end-gain already.

Timing

Hesitation and eagerness are both absent from a gesture that is properly timed. Here we must look again at the relationship of inhibition to time and speed.

The main purpose of inhibiting is to give you the opportunity to make a choice. To inhibit is to ask: Am I aware of what I am about to do? Do I really want to react in my habitual way? What alternatives do I have? Which do I prefer? Are my preferences dictated by habit, by default, or by choice?

Inhibition does not necessarily mean to take time to act, or to act slowly, or not to act altogether. Experienced Alexandrians can ask themselves all the questions I have proposed in a flash of a second. They can also ask themselves these questions at the very same time that they move, sing, play, walk, or speak. Alexander's scheme of conception, inhibition, direction, and action does not imply that you conceive *or* inhibit *or* direct *or* act. As you sing the first half of a melody you already think of its second half and inhibit your habits of misuse accordingly; you conceive, inhibit, direct, and act all at the same time.

Nevertheless, in learning how to inhibit it is useful to choose a gesture—sitting down, striking a chord, singing a scale—and take a few moments before executing it. You conceive the gesture in your mind; you inhibit your motivations to end-gain; you direct the use of your whole self. Then you *decide* to act. Immediately you take this decision, act! In other words, give yourself time between conceiving a gesture and executing it ('Look before you leap'), but not between deciding to act and acting ('He who hesitates is lost').

Husler and Rodd-Marling address this issue in connection with singing, particularly with the 'attack' (the onset of vocalization):

All muscle movements (tensing exercises) should be practised as *rapidly* as possible *to begin with*, never *slowly and hesitatingly*. . . . [Rapidly executed contractions] remind the muscles, as it were, of their own existence, by-pass 'bad habits' (habitual kinds of fixity, for instance) and other deficiencies in the vocal organ.

. . . [These movements] must be produced, at first, not only *rapidly*, but *suddenly*, without forethought or deliberation, in order to avoid certain complications that invariably set in when training begins.[11]

We find Cornelius L. Reid in complete agreement:

It is necessary . . . that the transformation of the breathing mechanism into a sound-producing instrument be initiated instantaneously. To do so other than quickly only serves to introduce interfering tension. . . . *Involuntary* responses have to be encouraged, and the only way to accomplish this is through precision of attack. By responding quickly to the pitch, intensity and vowel pattern, without regard to quality *per se*, a real breakdown of a wrong coordinative process becomes a distinct possibility.[12]

Note that Reid insists both on the instantaneous 'transformation of the breathing mechanism into a sound-producing instrument' and on disregarding 'quality *per se*'. Upon deciding to act, act at once and without regard to the end result of your action. '[Do] not to look backward once the course is decided upon,'[13] said Bruce Lee. To eliminate hesitation and over-eagerness, then, you will need to time the onset of your actions precisely; not to anticipate their outcome; and to suspend judgements of right and wrong, so as to become truly objective.

Earlier I wrote that for you to become free you need to act without worrying about the outcome of your actions. In an Alexander lesson or in a music lesson, this entails your taking risks, above all the risk of losing your habitual control. When it comes to learning something new and different, there are a number of possible attitudes. Let us take ice-skating as an illustration.

There are people who are simply unwilling to learn it. There are people who circle the rink slowly, prudently, holding on to the railing around it, never falling but never progressing. There are people who take a fall and pick themselves up again with grim determination, until they 'get it right'. And there are people who fall and laugh, people who love the sensations of uncontrol and of letting go of themselves and of going wrong. I often say to my Alexander pupils that there is something wrong in a lesson if at least one of the participants—teacher or pupil—is not laughing. To achieve freedom, then, take a risk, lose your balance, go wrong—and have a great time!

In time you pass from wrong to right. This very passing is also exceedingly enjoyable. You can then have fun when you go wrong, as you pass from wrong to right, and, naturally enough, when you go right.

Finally, note that 'conscious guidance and control', in Alexander's expression, does not entail your wilfully controlling every aspect of your every action. Good use and self-awareness are not the result of all that you do, but rather of all that you *stop doing*. Rather than controlling action, think of allowing it to happen. Undo the misuses of your head, neck, and back, and much that is right, easy, and thoroughly enjoyable will follow of its own accord.

Part II
The Procedures

7 The Lesson

Education and Therapy

The Alexander Technique, like all other fields of human knowledge, is taught in as many different ways as there are different teachers. A teacher always brings her temperament, personality, and background to bear upon her understanding of the Technique. This is both inevitable and desirable. Walter Carrington, a senior teacher trained by Alexander himself, says:

I remember that Ethel Webb, F. M.'s secretary, used to say that there was only one Alexander Technique, and that was the technique taught by F. M. Alexander: in so far as the rest of us taught it, we weren't really teaching the same technique. I'd agree with that to a certain extent. For this reason it's not altogether possible to distinguish between the Alexander Technique and the person who practises it. With such an individual and personal thing it's bound to be like that.[1]

Nevertheless, there should be at least a few elements common to all serious Alexander teachers. After all, the Technique is founded upon well-defined principles that have a certain internal logic and that are demonstrably in accord with immutable natural laws. In reality the term 'Alexander Technique' has come to encompass a wide range of disparate, and at times downright contradicting, practices. It is not within the scope of this book to consider why this is so. Further, it would be impossible to do justice here to all the different styles of teaching that co-exist today. I will describe a few different lesson formats, and explain the rationale behind the Alexander procedures presented in the chapters that follow. Readers who encounter styles of teaching that depart significantly from what I propose here will have to decide themselves on the merits and demerits of these styles, and of my own.

The first aspect of an Alexander lesson is just what the word implies: it is a lesson, not a therapy session. The Alexander teacher and her pupil have a teacher–student relationship, not a therapist–client one.

It is true that the Technique, by creating the right conditions for the organism to heal and regenerate itself, has often been used, and with great success, in the treatment of a series of illnesses and diseases. It is also true that many pupils first seek the help of an Alexander teacher because of a specific pathological condition, and frequently one that has persisted despite traditional medical care.

This, however, does not change the fundamental character of the Alexander Technique. The aim of the Alexander teacher is to help the pupil activate and refine the use of a Nature-given endowment: the ability to inhibit and direct. The teacher never sets out to cure a specific disease; rather, she works on the use of her pupil's whole self. Since disease is often caused at least in part by misuse of the self, the changes in use entailed by a committed study of the Alexander Technique tend to bring about the healing of disease. We could say that healing is a side-effect of the Alexander Technique, and the healing that does take place is always a *self-healing*. The teacher does not take credit for the healing; simply put, she is not a healer, and her pupil is not her patient.

This is not mere semantics. The roles of patient and pupil are different. The pupil takes full responsibility for his own well-being. He remains fully active, even as he learns to remain apparently passive when faced with certain stimuli. As Sherrington said, 'to refrain from an act is no less an act than to commit one, because inhibition is co-equally with excitation a nervous activity.'[2] The Alexander pupil learns *to do nothing*, but this is quite a different kind of nothing from that of the patient under the surgeon's scalpel or the acupuncturist's needles.

Emotions

During Alexander lessons many pupils go through deep emotional turmoil. The teacher is an agent in such turmoil, and yet she must not take the place of counsellor or therapist. Nobody can be all things to all people, and teachers are no exception. A teacher has three choices in dealing with her pupils' emotions. The first is not to deal with them at all: to create some distance—let us call it the pedagogical space—between herself and the pupil, and to make it clear to the pupil that he is there to learn the Alexander Technique, not to undergo psychotherapy. Establishing this pedagogical space need not be traumatizing to the pupil; it suffices that the teacher behave with common sense and normal human decency.

The second choice is for the teacher to receive counselling training and combine her teaching of the Technique with actual counselling. This has obvious advantages, and less obvious drawbacks. Once the limits of the pedagogical space are breached, teacher and pupil risk losing sight of the actual goals of the Alexander Technique, *goals which may well diverge from those of psychotherapy.*

The third choice is for the teacher to encroach in the pupil's emotional life without having received professional training. This is unwise and should be avoided by both teacher and pupil.

In sum, the Alexander Technique deals best with emotions when it does so indirectly, through inhibition and direction. The pupil will always be better served by an educational, rather than therapeutic, approach. To inhibit is to decide, *for yourself*, how best to react in any given situation, and to have the ability to carry out your own decisions. There could be no greater source of individual empowerment and emotional well-being.

The Absence of Exercises

There does not exist a set of Alexander exercises in the traditional sense of the word. Alexander teachers see no value in the repeated performance of prescribed exercises: twenty squats a day, for instance. You may well do a squat during an Alexander lesson, but the benefit you derive from it is not in its execution, but in its preparation. 'It is not getting in and out of chairs even under the best of conditions that is of any value,' said Alexander; 'that is simply physical culture—it is what you have been doing in preparation that counts when it comes to making movements.'[3]

The basic Alexander procedure consists, very simply, in the teacher's giving you a stimulus, and your reacting to it. In a lesson you go in and out of chairs, squat, walk, or lift your arms, not to perfect these different activities but to examine your reaction to a given stimulus, to become aware of what you are doing, to inhibit end-gaining and misuse, and to direct your whole self. The processes of sensory awareness, inhibition, and direction that precede and accompany every movement are of paramount importance; the movement itself is incidental, a means to an end and not an end in itself.

This disturbs many beginner pupils who have come to believe in the value of exercise. It is unsettling to be told *not* to exercise, after being told the contrary on so many occasions. It is also much easier to exercise for a half-hour every day (perhaps in front of the television) than actually to think about how you react to events and to people around you. In truth exercising and the Alexander Technique have very little in common, although you can apply the Technique to all your favourite exercises, whether related to music-making or not. (I shall discuss the issue of exercises further in Chapter 16, 'Daily Practice'.)

Alexander summed up the essence of a lesson neatly. 'You are not here to do exercises,' he said, 'or to learn to do something right, but to get able to meet a stimulus that always puts you wrong and to learn to deal with it.'[4] I often say to my pupils that their reactions in any given situation may be either *normal*—like everybody else's, as they have always been—or *natural*—according to the laws of Nature, as they should ideally be. In the course of an Alexander lesson the teacher presents you with a series of stimuli, with the object of helping you react to them *naturally* rather than *normally*.

The Hands-on Approach

One of the defining characteristics of the Alexander Technique is the teacher's use of her hands. Early on in his teaching career, Alexander found that his pupils' faulty sensory awareness made it difficult, if not impossible, for them to understand what he meant, unless he used his hands. I have dwelled on this issue in Chapter 3, 'Sensory Awareness and Conception'.

Some Alexander teachers today claim that using the hands is a subtle form of end-gaining. Rather than giving the pupil an experience, they prefer to help him through the steps that Alexander took himself in order to arrive at the experience. This we may call the 'hands-off' approach. According to Patrick Macdonald, Alexander used to tell his students that 'if you will do what I did, you will be able to do what I do.'[5] This may be true in principle; in practice it would take a person of Alexander's insight, patience, and determination—a person of his genius—to succeed in breaking the vicious circle of faulty conception and faulty experience without the help of guiding hands. I shall return to this issue in Chapter 14, 'Working on Yourself'.

Throughout a lesson a teacher will use her hands continuously to touch and handle the pupil. An Alexander teacher has different training, methods, and objectives from those of an osteopath, a masseur, or a healer; consequently the *feel* of her hands is different as well.

The teacher has various aims when using her hands:

1. *to monitor what the pupil is doing.* In some instances the teacher can even tell what the pupil is *thinking.* It is not a matter of telepathy, of course; while touching the pupil the teacher feels his hesitation, eagerness, anticipation, hurry, discomfort, and anxiety, and can easily draw conclusions about the assumptions behind the pupil's reactions. Remember yet again: there is no separation between so-called body mechanics and so-called mental states.

2. *to prevent certain things from happening.* For example, by placing one hand under the chin of the pupil and the other on his skull, the teacher can prevent the pupil's head from contracting into his spine, at rest or in movement.

3. *to encourage some other things to happen.* For example, by skilfully pressing on the hips of a pupil who is standing up, the teacher can create a certain stability in the lower body, which allows for greater freedom of the upper body.

These different functions of the teacher's hands overlap quite naturally. It is hardly possible for the teacher to use her hands exclusively to monitor the pupil's movements without causing some immediate change in the pupil's awareness and consequently in his use. If I place my hands on your ribcage, for instance, you are likely to alter your breathing immediately, regardless of the intentions with which I touch you.

We can speak of the hands of an Alexander teacher as being healing, guiding, or goading. The healing touch soothes and reassures the pupil, helps the release of excessive tension, and sometimes relieves headache, backache, and other types of pain. This touch and its effects have gained the Alexander Technique many a grateful devotee. This, I think, can lead to serious misapprehensions about the nature of the Alexander Technique. Its primary purpose is not to heal or soothe, much less to make the pupil feel good, but to teach him to inhibit and direct, *even if this causes discomfort or pain.* I shall return to this presently.

The guiding touch gives support and energy to the pupil as he goes through the various movements the teacher requires of him. In Chapter 4, 'Inhibition', I suggested how a teacher might help a cellist with his vibrato; this was a good example of the guiding touch at work. The educational work of an Alexander teacher is strongly associated with this kind of manipulation. Its importance becomes evident when we accept the pervasiveness of faulty sensory awareness. It is the guiding touch that breaks the vicious circle of an incorrectly perceived experience colouring perception, and of muddled perception colouring and predetermining experience.

Finally, there is the goading touch. A pupil of Patrick Macdonald once said to him, 'You do not do things to me with your hands; they persuade me to do things for myself.' 'This', comments Macdonald, 'should be the aim of every teacher.'[6] Persuasion is the ideal way. Sometimes, however, it fails. Pupils often resist the flow of change. They have many reasons for this: misuse, the fear of losing control, or just plain old pig-headedness. These barriers must be overcome. Cornelius L. Reid wrote of fast work in singing lessons: 'In general, slow moving passages are used when the student is being *encouraged to think*, fast moving passages to *bypass his wrong thinking*.'[7] Goading hands, acting with calculated speed or insistence, or both, throw the pupil away from his limited and limiting conception of how things should go, and into the swirl of experience. Sudden, powerful insights can come out of this forced loss of control.

The 'Applications' Approach and Group Work

The working hypothesis of an Alexander teacher is that misuse of the whole self is the root cause of specific shortcomings or illnesses. Therefore, the best way to overcome *all* shortcomings is to work on the use of the self, and not on the shortcoming itself. The better you use your whole self on a general basis, the better you will use yourself on a particular basis. Improve your total co-ordination and you will automatically improve your music-making, your abilities at games and sports, your digestion, breathing, and circulation, your interpersonal skills, and so on. Leave your total co-ordination unchanged, and you are less likely to affect your activities positively.

Besides the logic of proceeding from the general to the particular, the more you have invested—personally, emotionally, professionally—in an activity, the harder it is to bring change to this activity. Good Alexander teachers take this into account, and use simple gestures from daily life (such as sitting and standing) to help you become aware of your habitual reactions and learn to inhibit and direct. In time, you can apply your knowledge of inhibition and direction to all activities, including music-making.

There are Alexander teachers who work on their pupils' outside occupations from the very start of the lessons. In view of my observations about misuse, this is a risky proposition, and it takes a very resourceful teacher and an equally responsive pupil to bring it off. To my mind the 'first principles' approach is more likely to succeed than the 'applications' approach. I shall discuss this issue further, and in connection with music-making, in Chapter 18, 'Norms and Deviations'.

Traditionally the Alexander Technique has been taught on a one-to-one basis. If you accept the reason for the hands-on approach—the ever-pervasive faulty sensory awareness—then the difficulty of teaching the Alexander Technique to groups becomes apparent. Alexander held strong views on the matter. He believed in the need for personal change on an individual, not collective, basis:

Reliable sensory appreciation cannot be given on the mass teaching principle or by precept or exhortation. This can only be done by individual teaching and individual work. Moreover, people who are massed together are apt to be governed by the 'herd instinct,' and we need to help man to evolve beyond that influence as soon as possible, and to this end we must have conscious and individual development.[8]

Learning the Technique resembles learning music. Private piano lessons, for instance, will always remain much more useful than group classes. In situations where individual lessons are impossible, however, group classes may do some good. Nevertheless, the budding pianist whose entire training has been limited to group classes cannot claim to know much about playing the piano; so with an Alexander pupil whose sole experience has been a few group classes.

Master-classes are another matter altogether. To perform for a teacher, before a group of peers, is obviously beneficial. Similarly, to observe others reacting to the stimuli of an Alexander lesson is greatly educative. Thanks to faulty sensory awareness, you may find it easier to see someone else's end-gaining and misuse than to see your own, learning about your own behaviour by comparison and inference. This is the main merit of Alexander group work. You will accomplish real personal change, however, by working on your own, rather than in a group.

The Positions of Mechanical Advantage

What happens, then, during an Alexander lesson? As I mentioned earlier, an Alexander teacher will often start her work with ordinary activities such as sitting and rising from a chair. Besides these and other simple movements of daily life, the Alexander teacher helps the pupil through a series of procedures based on what Alexander once called 'positions of mechanical advantage'. This is a confusing but useful term, and it would be worth our while to elucidate its meaning.

You will remember from Chapter 1, 'The Use of the Self', Alexander's dictum that 'There is no such thing as a right position, but there is such a thing as a right direction.' Sitting, standing, and lying down become right or wrong positions according to how you direct yourself within each position. If you *think up*, every position of yours becomes right; if you *pull down*, none of your positions can ever be right. It follows that the important thing for you to do is not to place yourself in any one position, but to be able to direct your whole self upwards regardless of position. The question, then, is how best to learn how to direct.

Alexander found that by manually guiding a pupil into certain positions—some habitual, others not—he was able to encourage him to send the right directions, and thereby make these positions 'right'. The merit of the procedure depends not on the pupil's assuming a particular bodily position, but on his learning to direct on a general basis. Indeed, in some of these positions the pupil will be quite uncomfortable *unless* he directs his whole self. Alexander called them 'positions of mechanical advantage'. The positions are a means to an end, more than ends in themselves. Learn to think up in a position of mechanical advantage—the monkey or the lunge, for instance—and you can think up anywhere, any time in your daily life.

I shall describe some of these positions of mechanical advantage that are typical of an Alexander lesson: the monkey, the lunge, the hands on the back of the chair, the whispered 'ah', and table work. Today Alexander teachers use dozens of other procedures, from creeping and crawling on the floor to sitting on saddles. Yet I feel justified in limiting my choices to the above procedures for many reasons:

1. All were developed by Alexander himself, and their collective worth is thoroughly time-proven.
2. They are practical procedures with universal appeal and immediate, direct applications. Each procedure addresses one or more requirements common to all human beings, and you need not be suffering from a rare condition to benefit from doing it.
3. They can all be observed, altered, improved, and refined by the dual process of inhibition and direction.
4. They can all be monitored and changed by a teacher using her hands on the pupil.
5. They are procedures of ordinary daily life, un-esoteric, and un-complicated, even if learning them may be a complex process. (I shall discuss the difference between complicatedness and complexity in Chapter 13, 'Combined Procedures'.)
6. They are relevant and useful to all practising musicians.
7. Taken together, they address virtually all the aspects of co-ordinating the whole self. If you can do all the procedures well, there is little that will be beyond your capabilities.

The above considerations may also help you decide on the worth of other procedures you might learn in your Alexander lessons. In Appendix B, 'Questions and Answers', I shall discuss some of the practicalities of an Alexander lesson: how many lessons you should take, how to find a teacher, and so on.

In Chapters 9–13 I shall describe in detail some of Alexander's procedures. Before we proceed, however, I should like to discuss breathing. Alexander's understanding of breathing is radically different from accepted wisdom. In the Technique there are no breathing exercises, yet every Alexander procedure affects breathing in some way. To appreciate this apparent paradox, we need to study the question in detail.

8 Breathing

Confusion

Early in his teaching career, Alexander was known by many as 'the breathing man'. Even today, laymen and others seem to think that the Technique is a method for better breathing. It is true that Alexander had a keen understanding of the importance of breathing, and that lessons in the Technique may mitigate or eliminate many so-called breathing problems. Alexander himself, however, held views on breathing that are in nearly complete contradiction with much of current practice, and to think of his work as a method of breathing is to misunderstand both the essence of the Technique and the nature of breathing itself.

In a two-volume, 1,600-page work on the physiology of breathing we read:

Surely no organ or system of the human body is at present completely understood anatomically or physiologically. It would be difficult, however, to single out one vital organ concerning which more has been written, on which more lively differences of opinion are still expressed in print, and of which more remains to be learned, than the mammalian lung.[1]

With the evidence produced from many sources, the external and internal intercostals have been considered either expiratory or inspiratory, both inspiratory and expiratory acting simultaneously and alternately, and, finally, only regulating the tension of the intercostal space.[2]

The 'lively differences of opinion' are readily apparent when two or more singers, for instance, discuss breathing. Their views may be as divergent as to be mutually exclusive. There are many reasons for this. First, thanks to faulty sensory awareness, what singers (and others) think that they do is often different from what they actually do. Second, because so many people breathe badly, what is called *normal* breathing ('according to a statistical average') is not necessarily *natural* breathing ('ideal'), and yet in discussion we tend to take one for the other. (I shall examine the distinction between 'normal' and 'natural' in Chapter 17, 'Aesthetic Judgements'.) Third, it is difficult to observe natural breathing:

> Truly spontaneous breathing is extremely difficult to study because psychological factors have a strong influence on the way we breathe. For example, individuals unaware of breathing commonly breathe at rest between 15 and 20 BPM [breaths per minute]. As respiratory test subjects they usually breathe more slowly, between 10 and 15 BPM. Experienced test subjects tend to breathe more regularly than untrained subjects. . . . But regularity does not necessarily imply spontaneity.[3]

Fourth, even when a lay observer has accurately felt or observed ideal breathing, he is likely to describe it using empirical language ('relying on experience or observation alone often without due regard for system or theory'—*Webster's Ninth New Collegiate Dictionary*). In other words, he describes a correct experience, correctly gauged, using incorrect words, thereby contributing to the reigning confusion. Some singers, for instance, speak of the diaphragm when they mean the abdominal muscles. 'Pedagogic procedures initiated with the express intent of pushing the diaphragm "up" or "in"', writes Cornelius L. Reid, 'mistake diaphragmatic action for abdominal muscular tension. What creates the illusion of diaphragmatic activity is that the abdominal wall is pulled inward during expiration, and consequently moves the abdominal contents upwards.'[4]

Direct Control of Breathing

Alexander rightly considered breathing an effect, not a cause. We may say that *breathing is a function of use*, and as such it is outside direct control. Surely this is the defining characteristic of Alexander's understanding of breathing, and it puts the Technique in downright opposition to all schools of direct control of breathing, as exemplified by yoga and by much contemporary vocal teaching. I am aware that many of my readers will disagree strongly. Breathing is so bound up with emotional identification that it is hard for most people to discuss it dispassionately. Yet the facts bear up Alexander's understanding of breathing. The free-thinking Reid and the collaborating duo of Frederick Husler and Yvonne Rodd-Marling have put forth watertight arguments for the correct relationship of cause and effect as regards breathing and singing. Their books have proved hugely controversial, yet their detractors, rather than disproving the points made by their writers, have resorted to *ad hominem* attacks such as 'He is crazy.' Alexander was fond of saying that 'it doesn't alter a fact because you can't feel it'.[5] We can expand the dictum to say that it does not alter a fact because you cannot understand it, nor because you can not accept it.

Alexander held yoga in low esteem. We need not repeat in full his assessment of it here. Suffice it to say that he regarded a yogi's ability to, for instance, stop the beating of his heart as 'a dangerous trickery practised on the body', and of the 'well-known system of breathing practised and taught by [yogis]' he said: 'It is, in my opinion, not only wrong and essentially crude, but I consider that it tends also to exaggerate those very defects from which we suffer in this twentieth century.'[6] (Although Alexander tended to dismiss other people's convictions rather too quickly, here he was hinting at a real difference between yoga and his technique. This difference will become clearer as the current discussion progresses.)

Husler and Rodd-Marling, in addressing the issue of breath control, refer to yoga more charitably. They make the point that yoga, to give it its due, is a philosophy more than a set of exercises, and to practise the exercises without immersing yourself fully in the philosophy would subvert the nature of the exercises. The outlook of a yogi is essentially religious, and difficult for a Westerner to grasp or sustain. Independently of metaphysical arguments, Husler and Rodd-Marling argue convincingly that breath control cannot of itself lead to vocal control: 'Is there any guarantee that a breathing organ so treated and manipulated [by breathing exercises] will produce a properly functioning voice? The answer, of course, is "no," or "breath gymnasts" [e.g. yogis] with some application in other spheres, would all of them be excellent singers. Needless to say they are not.'[7]

The notion of 'breath support' is closely linked with that of breath control. I believe that if we are to give up the latter (and the Alexander Technique compels us so) we must inevitably abandon the former. Let us examine, then, two contrasting views of breath support.

Breath Support

The *Penguin Medical Encyclopedia* articulates the traditional view:

Singing makes very special demands on breathing. The singer breathes as much as possible with his diaphragm, which contracts more rapidly than the intercostals, and is thus a better means of snatching a quick breath. But a more important part of singing is controlled breathing *out*, and again the diaphragm is a better mechanism than the intercostals. If a singer tries to breathe with his intercostals—i.e. from the ribs—he has to control the out-flow by constricting the throat (as in 'loading' the lungs for a cough), and this produces the strangled tone of a bad singer. But if he breathes in with his diaphragm he distends the abdominal muscles, which he can then balance against his diaphragm to regulate the out-flow. The stream can be a torrent or a trickle, and the larynx plays no part in its regulation; its muscles need to be used only to determine the pitch of the note.[8]

Reid, whose writings should be cherished by all musicians and Alexander teachers, discusses a number of fallacies regarding breath support in his *Dictionary of Vocal Terminology*. 'Vocal tone', he points out, 'is nothing more than pressure variations created by an oscillation movement of the vocal folds whose frequency determines pitch. It is a physical impossibility to "support" these vibratory patterns.'[9] In other words, 'support' is at best an image, a metaphor rather than an actual physical process.

The authors of the *Penguin Medical Encyclopedia* speak of the singer breathing 'with his diaphragm'. This implies that the singer consciously initiates his breath with the diaphragm. Yet, Reid points out, 'the diaphragm is without proprioceptive nerve endings, and therefore without sensation. Thus, it is impossible to exercise any control over diaphragmatic movement except through the reflexive act of breathing.'[10] Alexander wrote that 'in all these contractions and expansions [of the thorax], the floor of the cavity (diaphragm) plays its part, moving upwards or downwards *in sympathy* with the particular adjustment of the bony thorax'.[11] You do not breathe because you move the diaphragm. Rather, you move your diaphragm because you breathe.

As for the control of the out-breath, Reid again advances a contrary view: 'The amount of breath expenditure is regulated by 1) a narrowing of the false vocal cords . . . and 2) the size of the glottal opening, which, in turn, is determined by . . . registration.'[12] Husler and Rodd-Marling concur emphatically: '*A properly functioning larynx regulates and trains to a high degree (by means of the ear) the respiratory muscles needed in singing.*'[13] Giovanni Battista Lamperti, despite writing at length about good breathing as a precondition of good singing, admits that 'finally the voice controls the breath—not the reverse'.[14]

The concept of breath support, concludes Reid,

leads to a self-conscious awareness of the body, confuses ends with means, and overlooks the fact that in an ideal technique all of the muscular systems involved are in equilibrium, which means that they are self-supporting. . . . The real question . . . [is] improving the co-ordinate relationship of a highly complex system of laryngeal muscles, which lies beyond volitional control. No known system of 'breath support' addresses itself to this problem.[15]

Michael McCallion, who based his *Voice Book* in large part on his Alexander studies, states that 'the whole question and practice of support is a vexed one in the world of voice production'.[16] Nevertheless he manages a useful definition of support: 'To put it simply, it is the refusal to collapse.'[17] Seen in this light support is not something you do, but something *the contrary of which you inhibit*—a non-doing rather than a doing.

We are almost ready to return to Alexander's understanding of breathing. First, however, consider this excerpt from Richard Miller's tome on 'national tonal preferences':

Appoggio is the term used [by the Italian school] to sum up the kind of muscular co-ordination on which the Italian system of breath management is based. . . . *Appoggio* embraces a total system in singing which includes not only support factors but resonance factors as well (witness such terms as *appoggiarsi in testa* and *appoggiarsi in petto*). With reference to breath management for the singing instrument, *appoggio* encompasses the interrelationship of the trunk and neck, combining and balancing them in such an efficient way that the function of any of them is not violated through the exaggerated action of another.[18]

Appoggio, then, is a 'total system', of which breathing is but an aspect. Reid clarifies matters further: 'It is true that when all of the muscular activities involved are in equilibrium one is aware of the body being in a comfortable, poised condition and of the voice being "supported."'[19] But this feeling of support is an end result of good singing, not the process by which you improve your voice—an effect not a cause. We can now turn to Alexander's views.

Breathing, Use, and Misuse

In Alexander's conception, the whole of breathing, good or bad, 'supported' or 'unsupported', is an effect, not a cause:

We say that a person is a 'bad breather,' or that he 'breathes imperfectly.' But we must remember that this so-called 'bad breathing' is only a symptom and not a primary cause of his malcondition, for the standard of breathing depends upon the standard of general co-ordinated use of the psycho-physical mechanism. What we ought to say, therefore, in such a case is not that a person 'breathes badly,' but that he is badly co-ordinated.[20]

The act of breathing is not a primary, or even a secondary, part of the process. . . . As a matter of fact, given the perfect co-ordination of parts as required by my system, breathing is a subordinate operation which will perform itself.[21]

Breathing straddles the line between voluntary and involuntary bodily functions. Reid points out that 'in common with all such systems, the following rule applies: if but one member of a complex muscular system is involuntary, all members of the system must be treated as though they, too, were involuntary'.[22] It will be easier to understand Alexander's view of breathing if we examine in detail the misuses of somebody who makes breathing primary and voluntary, rather than subordinate and involuntary.

Ask somebody to 'take a deep breath'. Most people will subject themselves to a series of misuses that could in no way enhance their breathing. These misuses are exaggerated by the performance of the exercise, but are equally present, albeit in a lesser degree, in most people most of the time: in movement or at rest, while speaking or while silent, in rehearsal or in performance, in a yoga class or in a physiotherapist's room. Most people 'suck air into the lungs to expand the chest' by gasping or sniffing; tense and shorten the neck, and depress the larynx; raise the upper chest and the shoulders to inhale, and collapse the chest to exhale; and hollow the back and protrude the abdomen.

Gasping and sniffing are nearly universal. You can check this for yourself by listening to radio or television announcers, singers and other musicians, people who speak to you, even the outgoing message in your own answering machine. Sniffing in air through the nose is both unnecessary and harmful. Alexander pointed out that it causes the collapse of the alae nasi, and that 'it also tends to cause congestion of the mucous membrane of the respiratory tract on the sucker system, setting up catarrh and its attendant evils, such as throat disorders, loss of voice, bronchitis, asthma, and other pulmonary troubles'.[23]

Of pulling the head back and down and crowding the larynx, Alexander wrote that it 'is undoubtedly the greatest factor in the causation of throat troubles, especially where professional voice-users are concerned'. He mentions the abnormally deranged intra-abdominal pressure, the increase in 'the intra-thoracic pressure, [which] dams back the blood in the thin-walled veins and auricles and hampers the heart's action', and the consequences of a depressed larynx on the freedom of the tongue, which is attached to it, and on the 'adequate and correct opening of the mouth for the formation of the resonance cavity necessary to the vocalization of a true "Ah." '[24]

Understanding the mechanics of inspiration may help you undo some of your breathing habits and the misuse they engender. Alexander wrote:

Inspiration is not a sucking of air into the lungs but an inevitable instantaneous rush of air into the partial vacuum caused by the automatic expansion of the thorax.[25]

If the thorax is expanded correctly the lungs will at once be filled with air by atmospheric pressure, exactly as a pair of bellows is filled when the handles are pulled apart.[26]

It is not necessary . . . even to think of taking a breath; as a matter of fact, it is more or less harmful to do so.[27]

This account of inspiration is centuries old. The image of the bellows is a recurrent one. Leonardo da Vinci referred to the motion of the intercostal muscles of respiration, and said that 'since there is no vacuum in nature, the lung which touches the ribs from within must necessarily follow their expansion, and the lung, therefore, being like a pair of bellows, draws in the air in order to fill the space so formed'.[28] 'The lungs are not expanded because they are filled with air, but they are filled with air because they are expanded,'[29] wrote Francisco Sylvius de la Boë in 1660.

Alexander pointed out that most people, when practising breathing exercises, 'have one fixed idea—viz., that of causing a *great expansion* of the chest—whereas its proper and adequate *contraction* is equally important. There are, indeed, many cases in which the expiratory movement calls for more attention than the inspiratory.'[30]

Indeed, the expansion of the chest that causes inspiration ought to occur reflexively—a point made nicely by Huster and Rodd-Marling: 'The singer who breathes out according to the laws of nature will have little difficulty in breathing in properly.... Once the air has been expelled the diaphragm automatically switches over to breathing in, a process that needs no attention or conscious effort; either, indeed, would be more likely to disturb this perfectly natural control.'[31]

People sometimes try to expand the chest and increase the intake of breath in order to alleviate the multiple symptoms, physical and psychic, of a perceived lack of breath. Yet the effects of hyperventilation, or overbreathing, are if anything worse than those of underbreathing. These effects include 'tenseness, tremors or occasionally tetany [muscle spasms] on the one hand and abnormal sensations such as numbness, deadness or "pins and needles" on the other ... hyperactivity, tension, emotional sweating and instability, and various visceral disturbances of heart, gut and bladder ..., dizziness, faintness, visual disturbances and altered states of consciousness'.[32] 'Hyperventilation acts by blowing off excessive quantities of carbon dioxide.... A low level of carbon dioxide *per se*', however, 'does not necessarily cause symptoms'; it is 'short-term fluctuations ... which are the hallmarks of the chronic hyperventilation syndrome'.[33] To do too little, to do too much, and to fluctuate from one to the other, then, are all harmful.

'If you allow your ribs to move, as Nature intended,' wrote Patrick Macdonald, 'you will breathe properly. What you have to learn is to let them move. Let is the operative word.'[34] This applies to both inhalation and exhalation, which, Alexander wrote, 'should be a controlled movement which *allows* the air to escape, not a special effort to "drive" it out'.[35] The most important thing about breathing, then, is not to *do* it, but to allow it to happen of its own. Ideally, 'breath "takes itself" rather than having to be taken'.[36] Let us now consider how.

What not to Do

The practical consequence of Alexander's understanding of breathing is that you do *nothing* to alter breathing *directly* in an Alexander lesson. There are no exercises in which you are asked to change the mechanics or the speed of your breathing, to count while you breathe in or out, to hold your breath or force it out, and so on. Instead, you must first clear your mind of all preconceived ideas you may have about breathing. With the help of a teacher, accept that your sensory awareness may be faulty. Become aware of your habitual misuses. Then, stop misusing yourself—and let your breathing right itself.

Husler and Rodd-Marling conclude their chapter on breathing with an extensive list of inhibitory instructions (exhorations to *stop doing* or *not to do*) that are in complete agreement with Alexander's views on breathing. They are in the main: do not practise breathing mechanically; do not pump yourself full of air before singing a phrase; do not hold or hoard air; do not breathe in deliberately; avoid breathing exercises without the contribution of the voice; avoid breathing systems that distort your figure.

We may summarize all good breathing advice thus: (1) stop constricting your breathing; (2) stop forcing your breathing. Stated otherwise, inhibit overbreathing, and inhibit underbreathing. 'Prevent the things you have been doing', said Alexander, 'and you are half way home.'[37]

Manuals for wind and brass instruments, like books on singing, usually contain advice on how to breathe properly. Most writers advocate direct, as opposed to indirect, control of breath. A few times, however, the advice given is on the right track. Consider the following excerpt from a book on trumpet playing: 'It is hoped that the advanced student practices good posture while playing, but the beginning student must remember that it is virtually impossible to obtain a good breath and dispose of it correctly unless the body is erect, whether in a sitting or standing position.'[38]

Substitute 'use' for 'posture', and the advice improves considerably. Now, it is true that good use of the self is a *necessary condition* for you to obtain a good breath and dispose of it. But it also happens to be *sufficient* for good breathing! Good breathing is simply a characteristic of good use. Achieve good use, and you will become a 'good breather' automatically.

Since all the procedures outlined in this book affect use, they all bear upon breathing too, but indirectly only. Prominent among the procedures is the whispered 'ah', which may seem like a breathing exercise to you. It is not, but you will find out about it in due course.

Finally, let us admit that some people have benefited from working on their breathing consciously and conscientiously. All the same, they might have learned more, better, and faster by working on their use instead, and leaving breathing alone. Let us remember, too, those whose difficulties have increased because of their deliberate breathing exercises. The very least that can be said in favour of Alexander's non-doing approach was best said by Alexander himself: 'If I went to a man to take singing lessons, it wouldn't matter what he taught me, he couldn't injure me.'[39]

9 *The Monkey and the Lunge*

The Monkey

As I wrote earlier, styles of teaching the Alexander Technique vary from teacher to teacher. Also, a good teacher varies her own approach according to the needs of each pupil. Therefore, we cannot say that there is a standard Alexander lesson. If there is a basic, universal Alexander procedure, however, it is the one known as the monkey, as many teachers teach it to many of their pupils.

The monkey is a position of mechanical advantage. It co-ordinates the use of the back and legs, a precondition to improving other parts of the self, such as the upper limbs or the lips, tongue, and jaw. The monkey is also simpler and somewhat easier to perform than the hands-on-the-back-of-the-chair or the whispered 'ah' (which I describe in the chapters that follow). It is, therefore, logical to learn it before other procedures.

The monkey is an apt way of examining the issues of tension, relaxation, balance, posture, position, movement, control, inhibition, and direction. Besides being effective in developing co-ordination on a general basis, the monkey is useful when you need to lower yourself: to wash your face, to iron clothes, to sign a cheque on a shop counter, to pick an object off the floor, and so on. Since there are countless such situations in daily life (and in the life of a practising musician), the monkey is indeed an indispensable co-ordinative procedure.

Here and in other chapters, I describe a procedure, its pitfalls, and its applications. Before you decide to dispense with the help of a qualified teacher in learning the monkey, consider the following observations.

1. In all likelihood, your sensory awareness is faulty. By yourself, you risk performing monkeys badly; indeed, you may even harm yourself. The teacher assesses your needs, demonstrates and explains the procedure, guides you with her hands, gives you objective feedback about your performance, and advises you on how to perform on

your own. Written instructions cannot take the place of a teacher, regardless of how clearly the instructions are written and how intelligently you read them.

2. You may need to approach the monkey, or any other procedure, differently from somebody else. It is impossible to set a formula for all. Also, your own needs and abilities change from lesson to lesson. The monkeys you perform today may bear little resemblance to the monkeys you perform in three weeks' time.

3. During an Alexander lesson, the teacher helps you into a monkey without your having made a priori assumptions about what a monkey is or should be. In other words, you will not really know what a well-performed monkey feels and looks like until after the event.

4. The real nature of the procedure is one of co-ordination, not of position. Learn the principles of co-ordination in the process of doing monkeys, and you can apply the principles to all positions. If you treat monkeys as positions to be held for a few minutes a few times a day, you will have missed their point entirely.

Habitually, to lose height and to lean over (e.g. to pick an object up off the floor) most people bend their backs and stoop. The human back has a certain innate flexibility. With training it can become very pliable indeed. This does not mean that bending the back is beneficial or natural. Keep two points in mind. First, that which 'feels natural' to you may not be 'according to the laws of nature', a point I shall clarify in Chapter 17, 'Aesthetic Judgements'. Second, you may derive some benefit in the short term from bending your back—a feeling of so-called relaxation, for instance—but at a high price in the long term. Give up bending your back, then, even though it may seem natural and make you feel good. We will come back to this point later.

To go into a monkey, stand up and place your feet at shoulder width or slightly wider, pointing your toes outwards slightly. Bend your knees slightly. Now lean forwards from the hip joints. Practical need should determine where you place your feet and how far you bend your knees or lean forwards. Normally you should become able to do monkeys of any height with equal ease.

Simple as it sounds, the monkey is difficult to perform to perfection. The main reason for this lies in the antagonism between direction and movement. Most people pay more attention to the movement that sets up the position than to the directions that would make the movement free. Your body moves down and forwards in space when you bend your knees and lean over, and yet you should carry on directing it upwards and backwards before, during, and after the movement. In other words, you should *think up* to bend your knees and *think up* to lean forwards.

Misuses of the Self in the Monkey

Neglecting the primacy of direction over movement and position causes a series of misuses. You will need to become aware of them and to inhibit them. Here follows a list of *things not to do*. If this approach strikes you as unduly negative, keep Alexander's words in mind: 'Prevent the things you have been doing and you are half way home.'[1]

- When first bending the knees, do not let the chest drop forwards; do not let the pelvis go forwards; do not stick your bottom backwards. The torso should stay upright, undisturbed by the bending of the knees.
- Do not let your knees come inwards, towards one another. 'Knees forwards and away' is a perennial direction when using the legs—that is, forwards in space, away from the hips, and away from one another.
- Do not tighten your toes at any time.
- Do not stiffen your arms or hold your breath. Both are obviously unnecessary when you bend your knees.
- When you lean forwards in space, *the head should lead and the body follow*, rather than the other way around. (Please refer to Chapter 2, 'The Primary Control', for illustrations of this important principle.) To keep the relationship between the head and the back constant, the neck needs muscle tone. Remember, 'free' does not mean 'floppy'. Do not let your head go back and down (contracting into your spine), or forwards and down (hanging towards your chest).
- When leaning forwards, keep lengthening and widening the back; do not slump and do not hollow the back. At first this will seem difficult to do. You may feel that you are losing your balance and about to fall forwards or backwards, and you may attempt to keep your balance by contracting various parts of your body. Such feelings of imbalance arise both during successful and unsuccessful

executions of a monkey, and you will need to come to terms with them.

- A beginner often looks down at the ground while leaning forwards. This normally causes the head to sink somewhat, which you should avoid. All the same, do not fix your eyes in any one position and do not stare: a visual blank is always symptomatic of a mental blank. The eyes should be alert and mobile at all times, and able to move independently of the head. If I ask you to drop your eyes you need not drop your head, and if I ask you to look upwards you need not tip your head backwards, into the spine.

Variations

1. It is useful to perform monkeys while leaning with your back against a wall. This helps you keep your balance as you lean forwards. Stand with your back against a wall. Place your feet at shoulder width or slightly wider, a few inches away from the wall, the toes pointing out slightly. Make sure that you are pointing back against the wall with your back, *not your head*, which should remain clear of the wall. It is the spine which supports the head, not the wall. Bend your knees slightly. Then lean forwards slightly, all the while keeping your bottom against the wall. Let your arms hang freely by the side of your trunk. Here I remind you once more that without the 'upward thought along the spine' this whole procedure is useless. This thought and its attendant feeling are indescribable and are best learned with the help of a good Alexander teacher.

Experiment with the following variables when executing monkeys, both free-standing and against the wall:

- the distance between feet and their angle to each other;
- the degree to which you bend your knees;
- the degree to which you lean forwards;
- the speed of each phase of the movement.

Obviously, these variables are independent of one another. With feet wide apart, for instance, you may bend the knees and lean forwards a lot; with the feet close together, you may bend your knees a lot and not lean forwards at all. These are only two examples. There is infinite variation in the monkey. What characterizes an Alexander procedure is not a position of bodily parts in space but the directions (or tendencies) that these parts may have, one in relation to the other and each in relation to the whole. You should be able to do every combination and variation with equal ease. Note that a very low monkey becomes a squat.

2. There are many different ways of going into a monkey. The easiest is bending the knees first, then leaning forwards. It highlights the different directions and tendencies that you need to get into a monkey, and lessens the likelihood of your losing your balance as you lower yourself. Experiment with going into a monkey by first leaning forwards, then bending the knees; in a single gesture, without separating the bending of the knees from the leaning forwards of the trunk; from sitting; from a lunge.

3. The monkey is an excellent preparation for sitting down. In effect, most people sit down by first going through a rather badly executed monkey. (They are not aware of this.) Experiment with passing from a monkey (in its infinite variety of degrees) to sitting down, always keeping in mind that to apply the Technique successfully you should look as if you are not applying it all. Finally, experiment with going from sitting into a monkey. Not very easy, and nearly useless, but good fun.

Applications

A well-executed monkey is a position of great stability and strength. The legs give much-needed support to the whole body, and the torso becomes firm and elongated. Breathing is enhanced, as there is a natural tendency for the back to widen and the ribcage to expand. Because the legs are supporting the whole body, the upper limbs need not concern themselves with keeping balance, and are free to engage in whatever activity the situation demands of them.

Most healthy children, particularly very young ones, go naturally in and out of monkeys as they play. Brandon Lee, Bruce Lee's son, demonstrates perfect poise in a wide-footed, deep monkey (Fig. 7). Note that his monkey is vigorous and dynamic; in it Brandon displays necessary tension rather than relaxation. Older children can also be taught to do monkeys with ease and elegance. In Fig. 8 Alexander, placed in a lunge, works with a young girl for whom a monkey seems entirely natural.

Well-co-ordinated adults use monkeys in a variety of settings. Look at the picture of Wilhelm Furtwängler skiing (Fig. 9). He is bending the knees and leaning forwards from the hips, while keeping the back straight and the head well poised on top of his spine. Clearly 'his head leads, his body follows' as he skis downhill.

The picture of the cellist Aldo Parisot teaching a young pupil (Fig. 10) illustrates how you may express enthusiasm and passion while retaining—nay, enhancing—your upward thought. The pupil would do well to imitate this ability of Mr Parisot's. Both Parisot and Furtwängler demonstrate how well-co-ordinated men and women use themselves well in every situation: in music-making, in sports, in daily living. Were you to learn how to do monkeys to principle, all aspects of your use and functioning would benefit, not least your music-making.

It is useful for a musician to practise his instrument (or his singing) while in the monkey. Take, for instance, an oboist who habitually sways his whole body and bends his legs as if choreographing his own playing. This swaying is but a squandering of precious energy, which is being dispersed rather than directed into actual music-making. The effects of this waste of energy are numerous: greater tiredness at the ends of rehearsals and concerts, possible rhythmic inaccuracies and fingering difficulties, an unfocusing of the sound, both in its quality and in its projection in the concert-hall, and seasickness in fellow musicians and in discriminating members of the audience.

Undisciplined and excessive moving about on stage is typical of many musicians who perform standing up: wind and upper-string soloists, singers, conductors, and so on. It is often symptomatic of technical deficiencies rather than interpretive choices. William Primrose, the great violist, said of excessive swaying:

I sometimes see a lot of bobbing and weaving on the part of the soloist, which disturbs me terribly. In contrast to this shadow-boxing manner, Heifetz and Kreisler were ideal examples of great distinction on the platform, great aristocracy. . . . With a few [musicians], [this weaving] becomes almost a vulgarity. The facial expressions and the sinuous movements and gyrations simulate those of a belly-dancer. Excessive movement is usually a part of a person's nature, and if ingrained, it is very difficult to stop. It may be unconscious, or to an extent it can come from the instinct to show off, I suspect. I am not sure if there might not be an influence from current rock performing stars. Sometimes I can draw a student up sharp by saying, 'Look, with your moving about in that way, you have to

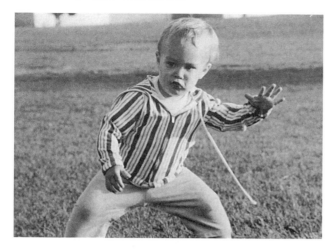

FIG. 7. The young Brandon Lee

FIG. 8. Alexander, in a lunge, teaches the monkey to a child

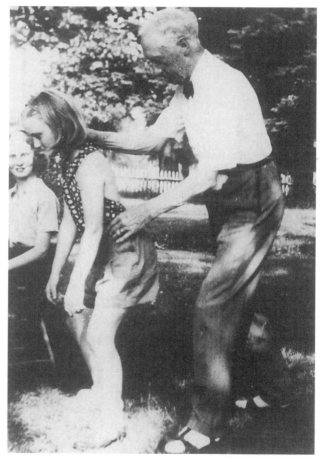

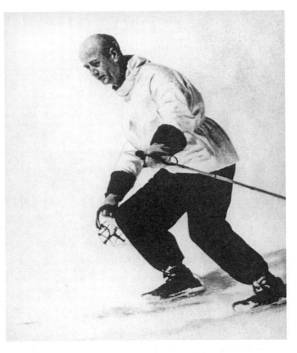

FIG. 9. Wilhelm
Furtwängler

FIG. 10. The cellist
Aldo Parisot teaching
a young student

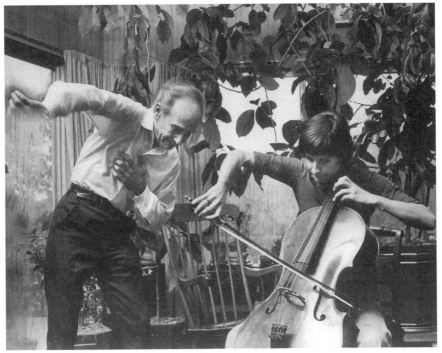

remember that the F-holes are on different planes all the time. The tone is always coming out at a different angle, which is undesirable. Also, from my standpoint, your gyrating is unsightly.'[2]

Richard Shepherd Rockstro wrote a comprehensive treatise on the flute, drawing on many historical sources. Of a flautist moving on stage, he writes:

The player should stand or sit as still as possible; there must be no swaying of the head or the body in cadence with the music, nor must there be any of the ungainly and ridiculous rolling and contortions too often substituted for musical expression. A true musician will endeavour to produce an effect by his artistic rendering of the music of which he is the exponent; not by any acting or attitudinizing.[3]

An excellent way to stop this gyrating is to put the offender in a monkey position, perhaps with his back against the wall. As I have remarked, the monkey enhances the use of the legs and of the back, and gives stability and solidity to the whole body. The results of playing or singing in a monkey are often startling. The sound becomes more focused, evenly produced and projected; rhythm and articulation become reliable, rubatos convincing; the musician's appearance becomes professional and authoritative. (You need not give a public performance in a monkey: use it as a learning tool in the practice room.)

The Lunge

The lunge is a variation on the monkey. Again the body is lowered in space, but now the feet are usually placed asymmetrically and one of the legs is bent, the other straight. Otherwise, its basic principle is the same as the monkey's: bending the joints (of hips, knees, and ankles) while keeping the relationship between head, neck, and back constant—the neck always free, the head leading forwards and up, and the back lengthening and widening.

Within a lunge there is infinite variation of movement and relativity of parts. The lunge can be thus adapted to a huge number of practical tasks, both in daily life and in music-making.

There are numerous ways of getting into a lunge. I shall start by describing the most formalized of these ways, because it contains the greatest number of opportunities for inhibiting, directing, and *thinking up* against a habitual reaction of misuse. I describe a *left lunge*. A right lunge requires symmetrical steps.

1. Stand up and place your feet side by side.
2. Put the heel of the left foot on the hollow of the right foot—that is, advance the left foot forwards slightly and put the left foot at an angle of about forty-five degrees to the right foot.
3. Turn your head and trunk so that you are facing in the same direction as your left toes.
4. Lift your left knee up in the air, so that your foot is clear of the floor.
5. Lean forwards and let the left foot drop, away from the right foot.
6. Bend your left knee slightly.
7. Lean your trunk forwards, from your hips.

This particular form of the lunge is useful because you can perform and repeat each step independently of all the others, making it easier for you to prevent the many instances of misuse that each step may cause. Remember Frank Pierce Jones's definition of the means-whereby principle: 'The co-ordinated series of intermediate steps which must be accomplished in order to attain an end. The means-whereby principle is the recognition in practice that these intermediate steps are important as ends in themselves'.[4]

Misuses of the Self in the Lunge

Several of the misuses which afflict a badly co-ordinated monkey are also evident in a lunge. I shall not list them all again. Instead, I consider each of the intermediate steps, and highlight new misuses which you and your teacher will work on together.

1. When you put your feet wide apart or close together again, do not let your head twist in any direction (sideways, forwards, or backwards). When you move your body, inertia may well cause the head to move as well (as in whiplash, for instance), but you should have enough muscle tone in your neck to prevent this needless and harmful movement. As you shift your balance from leg to leg, do not twist your torso or your hips. Contracting the torso or swinging the hips is

a compensating mechanism for an apparent loss of balance. Patrick Macdonald quotes Peter Scott, a very fine Alexander teacher: 'For anyone who is inclined to lose their balance when standing, I can only advise that proper standing seems to be an activity more like swimming than a mechanical achievement of stability.'[5] Aim not to keep your balance at all moments, but rather to be able *to lose your balance without losing the lengthening of the spine.* Remember, too, that the Technique gives you a new (and more natural) balance, and for you to learn it you need to lose your old balance first. If you find yourself dragging your feet as you open and close your legs, you are probably making your body heavy. Think up away from your feet, 'let the head lead and the body follow', and you will find it easier to move lightly and elegantly.

2. When you put the heel of one foot next to the hollow of the other, take care again not to swing the body unnecessarily (in an attempt to catch your balance), and do not turn your trunk together with the leg. Throughout the lunge you should aim for an independence of bodily parts, so that the movement of a part (a leg or a foot, for instance) does not disturb the arrangement of the other parts (the head and neck, the back, the arms, etc.).

3. When you turn the torso in the direction of your turned-out toes, keep the relationship between your head, neck, and back constant, and avoid twisting your chest or contracting your torso.

4. Most people find it difficult at first to lift a knee without upsetting the balance of the whole body. Lifting the knees is necessary in walking, in climbing or descending stairs, in putting your foot up a step to tie your shoelaces, and so on. You may wish to steady yourself at first by gently touching a wall or a chair as you lift your knee. Make this only a temporary measure to help you inhibit misuse; it should not become a crutch.

5. Leaning forwards and placing the front foot down cause problems for most pupils, who tend to land heavily on their front foot, with an unpleasant thud that reverberates throughout the whole body. Like all misuse, this denotes a deficiency in *thinking up along the spine.* Make sure not to reach forwards with the foot, which causes the lower back to hollow. Instead, lead forwards with the back, and use your front foot to stop yourself from falling.

6. When you land on your front foot, the leg will naturally be bent (at the hip, knee, and ankle). Once you find yourself in this position, you may bend and unbend your front knee at will. Here you risk

swaying your hips, hollowing your lower back, and throwing your head back by inertia. As in all other situations, 'the head should lead, the body should follow'. Make sure not to lead with your hips as you bend your knee. In this position, two tendencies have to be checked: an excessive relaxation of the leg, which causes wobbliness and insecurity, which in turn causes the neck to tighten as a compensating mechanism, and an excessive rigidity of the joints, which causes lack of freedom and mobility. Bending and unbending the front knee in this position is useful for many reasons. Movement may enhance flexibility; a dynamic balance is often easier to achieve and maintain than a static one; and to move is to give yourself a stimulus possibly to go wrong, which creates the opportunity for yet more inhibiting and directing.

7. Finally, when you lean your trunk forwards from your hip you create the same possibilities for misuse that you did in the similar movement in the monkey: slumping, curving, or hollowing the back, moving the head by inertia, tightening your shoulders and arms, constricting your breathing, and so on.

We shall turn to the lunge's practical applications shortly. But from the above observations it should become clear that the lunge, besides being useful in daily life, is an extremely valuable procedure for learning how to inhibit misuse and send directions to the whole self. Let us always keep in mind Alexander's saying: 'There is no such thing as a right position, but there is such a thing a right direction.' Devoid of direction, as a mere position in space, the lunge has no more merit than any other bodily posture. Yet, if you inhibit the myriad misdirections possible in a lunge, you will have placed yourself in a 'position of mechanical advantage', and you will have learned something much more valuable than simply a useful body position.

Variations

As with all Alexander procedures, there is not a single, fixed way of lunging. The lunge, like the monkey, must become easy, natural, spontaneous, automatic even; there should be nothing formal or artificial about it. The step-by-step lunge that I have described is useful in the wealth of opportunities it affords for avoiding end-gaining and for inhibition. Yet simply to take a step forwards and to the side is to lunge too.

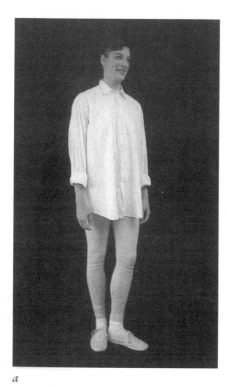

a

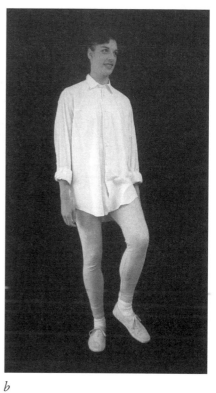

b

FIG. 11. The lunge

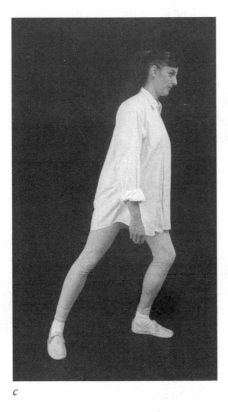

c

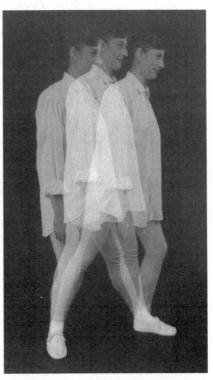

d

You can easily combine one or more of the steps I have described. To give but an example, you can put your feet together and your left heel in your right hollow, and turn your head and trunk in a single gesture. You can also experiment with several different variables as you lunge: the distance between the feet and the angle between them, the height to which you lift your knee, the degree to which you bend your knees, the inclination of the trunk, the speed at which you lunge, and so on.

It is easy to get both in and out of a lunge. Remember Heinrich Neuhaus's definition of a good position: 'one which can be altered with the maximum of ease and speed'. Study the pictures of an Alexander pupil going into a lunge and moving backwards and forwards while staying in a lunge (Fig. 11a–d). It is easy to go into a lunge and to move within one—as long as you think up to do it. The lunge is very stable, but neither rigid nor fixed. There are at least five distinct ways of going from a left lunge to a right lunge. Rather than describing them, I shall leave it for you to discover them for yourself.

Place yourself in a lunge with your feet close together: this is an excellent all-purpose standing position. It is in fact easier to think up and to energize the whole organism when the feet are in this asymmetrical position. With the feet parallel, you will tend to push the pelvis forwards and hollow and shorten the back. (Alexander called this the 'Clubman's Stance'.) Besides the greater ease of pointing up along the spine, the narrow lunge affords liberty of movement as well. You can easily shift your body weight forwards and backwards (thereby relieving tiredness in the legs), take steps in any direction, lean forwards and backwards, bend downwards, go into a monkey, and so on. The lunge is useful as preparation for walking, dancing, or climbing up steps, as a position for standing up for long periods of time, in pushing heavy furniture around or lifting things up, as preparation for leaning over and reaching for objects that are not at arm's length, and in many other ways.

In the early stages of Alexander training, a pupil often feels that the monkey and the lunge are uncomfortable contrivances. He claims that he feels out of balance in a monkey, that his legs are too tense or too wobbly, that he would 'look funny' if he did a monkey in a public place. The effect of his combined arguments is to make him believe that the monkey is not natural.

As positions of mechanical advantage, the monkey and the lunge are not exclusive to the Alexander Technique. Well-co-ordinated people of all ages, in all cultures, go in and out of monkeys and lunges all the time, effortlessly and elegantly. Normal, healthy children play in monkeys; peoples that have been unaffected by the debauching effects of civilization—South American aborigines, the Masai—use monkeys for hunting, dancing, playing, and daily living; good skiers, ice-skaters, and wind-surfers do the monkey; master martial artists do monkeys and lunges. In every case the monkey and the lunge are contributing factors to healthy, efficient living.

This goes to prove that the monkey and the lunge are intrinsically natural, that is, innate to the human organism. They might *feel* unnatural to the badly co-ordinated pupil, but this is only a function of faulty sensory awareness. In due course every Alexander pupil passes from believing that it is unnatural to do monkeys to simply doing them *reflexively*—without apparent interference from the conscious mind.

The apparent complication of a lunge should not put you off. Alexander made a fine distinction between 'complex' and 'complicated', which I shall discuss in Chapter 13, 'Combined Procedures'. For the moment it suffices to say that the lunge is not complicated, although it requires a complex arrangement of body parts, the working of which is perfectly simple.

The end result of a committed study of the Alexander Technique is a seamless ease of movement and gesture. It is easy to go in and out of monkeys and lunges, and from one into the other; monkeys are good preparations for sitting down, lunges for walking. It means that sitting, standing, walking, climbing, leaning, bending, squatting can all flow each from the other.

Applications

Like the monkey, the lunge is used by children, athletes, performers, and many others. That the lunge is timeless can be seen in the bronze by Jacopo Alari Bonacolsi (Fig. 12). The sculpture itself dates from nearly 500 years ago; presumably it depicts a Roman youth of earlier times still.

Seigo Yamaguchi, a great aikido master, demonstrates the power of a stable yet dynamic lunge (Fig. 13). The lunge is not culturally determined; it follows from the logic of the very organism. Therefore it remains right and good in every culture, in every era: in Rome two

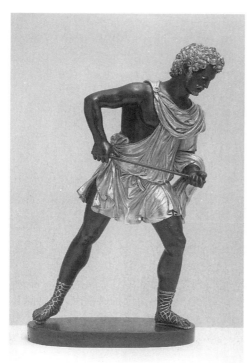

FIG. 12. Bronze by Jacopo Alari Bonacolsi (*c.*1460–1528)

FIG. 13. Seigo Yamaguchi and Christian Tessier

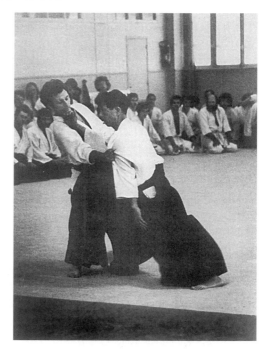

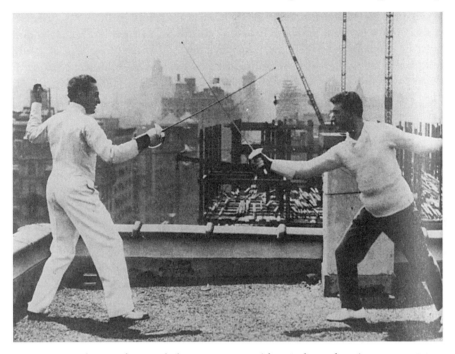

FIG. 14. Jascha Heifetz and the composer Isidor Achron lunging atop a New York skyscraper.

thousand years ago, in Japan, atop a New York City skyscraper (Fig. 14). See how Jascha Heifetz and the composer Isidor Achron fence in well-grounded lunges, leaning forwards and backwards as needed and thinking up before and during every movement. Heifetz's use was great at the violin and away from it. If you wish to emulate him, start by working on your lunges.

The close-footed lunge is an ideal posture for all musicians who perform standing up: woodwind soloists, upper-string players, conductors, Lieder singers, and so on. Keep in mind, however, that the word 'posture' does not imply a rigid body position, but a flexible, dynamic *relativity* of body parts. In the Alexandrian concept of 'position of mechanical advantage', the body is in a state of permanent, latent mobility which may be actualized at any moment, according to the needs of the music.

I should like to quote one authority on the applications of the close-footed lunge to flute playing:

If standing, the player should be well balanced on the legs, with the left foot advanced, and the weight of the body resting chiefly on the right hip. This position must be maintained without the least constraint. . . . These directions, carefully followed, will promote a very graceful attitude, which will be not less pleasing to the eye than the tone of the instrument will be agreeably soothing to the ear.[6]

Thus wrote Hotteterre-le-Romain in around 1700, advising flautists, oboists, and recorder players alike. A modern treatise on flute playing concurs: 'One foot should be a bit in front of the other to ensure balance.'[7] Compared with the later writer, Hotteterre-le-Romain may strike you as old-fashioned. But there is, I believe, more virtue in his advice, above all because of the use of the word 'attitude' in connection with the player's bearing.

You may argue that Hotteterre-le-Romain's advice sounds old-fashioned because it *is* old-fashioned: the 'graceful attitude' which is pleasing to the eye seems stiff to the modern musician. The lunge is not 'cool'. Patrick Macdonald wrote that during an Alexander lesson 'one of my students . . . said that he felt "old fashioned." I believe this to be a very good description of what one is likely to feel when the body's co-ordination is improving.'[8]

Bodily movement is natural and necessary in music-making. But the movements of a badly co-ordinated musician are ineffective and ungainly. Often they are determined not by a musical need but by habit, by technical insufficiencies, or by a desire to 'show off'. A musician who moves haphazardly or excessively while playing or singing may use the lunge both to become aware of these movements and to change them. Further, the lunge, well grounded as it is, contains the seeds of truly natural mobility. You need not worry that the lunge will stop your playing from being free. On the contrary: by co-ordinating all your motions (those that facilitate a technique as well as those that give flight to your expressivity) with the various movements that a lunge affords, you can make your playing freer than if you move willy-nilly.

The lunge is part of the foundation of technique for all bowed-instrument players. This may be clear for violinists, violists, and bass players, less so for cellists (who must by necessity sit down to play). Yet even a cellist's basic co-ordination is related to the lunge, thanks to the phenomenon of quadrilateral transfer, which we shall discuss in the next chapter.

Lunging, Walking, Sitting, and Standing

The close-footed lunge is a comfortable, stable, and well-balanced position for all-purpose standing. One of the reasons why it is a comfortable position is that it can be very readily altered. (Remember Heinrich Neuhaus's definition of a good position: one which can be changed with the greatest ease and speed.) You can go easily in and out of lunges, from lunges to monkeys, from left-footed lunges to right-footed ones, and from a static lunge into walking and vice versa. Simply put, right walking starts with right standing, and the close-footed lunge is useful as preparation for walking and as a resting-point in between steps.

Go back to my description of the various phases of the lunge, and you will see that at some point as you perform a lunge you find yourself standing on one foot, the other lightly raised and poised in front of you. Walking is not so much a matter of placing this raised foot down in order to propel yourself forwards as a matter of inclining your whole body forwards, from the rear ankle upwards, and using the raised foot to stop yourself from falling.

In other words, the primary source of the forward progress in walking is a movement of the body, not of the feet. Most people walk by leading their bodies with their feet, throwing the pelvis forwards and hollowing the back. Instead, see yet again that 'the head leads, the body follows', and walk up *off* each step, not down *into* each step.

The lunge can also be a preparation for sitting down. The Technique is a method not of 'right sitting and standing', but of improving your use in every conceivable situation. People who use themselves well can sit and stand in any way they please. As used during an Alexander lesson, the acts of sitting, standing, and lunging, although ends in themselves, are above all means to a greater end: the co-ordination of the whole self on a general and permanent basis.

Keep the above points in mind, then, and lunging and sitting will become positive, health-giving experiences. Stand in a close-footed lunge next to a chair, facing away from it. Let your neck be free, to let your head go forward and up, to let the back lengthen and widen, all together, one after the other. While still thinking up, let your hips move back in space and let your knees bend. If you bend your knees enough, sooner or later you will find yourself sitting down. To stand up, simply reverse the procedure.

If instead of directing upwards and bending your knees you give yourself the command to sit down, you will almost certainly misuse yourself. Think then of the means, not the end. And be willing to accept that learning to think up from a book is impossible.

10 *The Arms and Hands*

Introduction

A musician's use of his arms and hands is of paramount importance; on this we can all agree at once. Indeed, pianists, string players, and conductors, among others, spend much of their practice time examining and exercising their upper limbs. This is reasonable, considering the complex requirements of their music-making. Yet, if musicians neglect other aspects of their use, they risk lessening the efficacy of their upper limbs by their very efforts to improve them.

This undue preoccupation is unwittingly typified by the following definition of violin technique, given by a master teacher: 'Technique is the ability to direct mentally and to execute physically all of the necessary playing movements of left and right hands, arms, and fingers.'[1]

Most musicians would accept this definition. I shall discuss its flaws in Chapter 15, 'Technique'. For now it suffices to say that it fails to consider the use of the arms and hands in relation to the rest of the self. The purpose of this chapter is to establish such a relationship, all the while discussing in detail Alexander's views on the specific use of the arms and hands and seeing how a musician can put these views into practice.

We start with an experiment in observation. Because of faulty sensory awareness, it will be easier for you to get its point by performing it with somebody else.

Tell a friend to stand up, feet apart to shoulder width, and ask him to lift both his arms in front of him, to shoulder height, the elbows straightened and the palms facing down. If your friend's use is but average, he will pull his head back and down; lift his shoulders up and in, towards the neck; shorten his spine, narrow his upper back, and hollow his lower back; sway his upper body backwards; and stick his pelvis forwards. He is also likely to stop breathing and to stare vacantly in space, two common symptoms of misdirected 'concentration'.

Different people misuse themselves to different degrees, but the pattern I describe is nearly universal. It demonstrates that most people, when using their arms, interfere with the correct use of the head, neck, and back. Lifting the arms as I describe in my experiment is similar to what conductors, string players, pianists, trombonists, and all other musicians do in their music-making. We need, therefore, to find ways of using the arms that do not interfere with the Primary Control—better still, ways that positively enhance its workings.

Alexander developed such a procedure, and called it 'putting hands on the back of a chair'. Alexander teachers have many different ways of working on the arms and hands. I limit my discussion to Alexander's original procedure because it is comprehensive in its scope; the pupil who has mastered it will find that all other Alexandrian ways of examining and changing the use of the arms and hands cover familiar ground. Alexander described 'hands on the back of the chair' in detail in his second book, *Creative Conscious Control of the Individual*. Patrick Macdonald had much to say about it as well, and in this discussion I am indebted to both Alexander and Macdonald.

I would like to remind my readers that if they attempt this procedure on their own, without the help of a teacher's knowing hands, they are likely to run into all the usual difficulties created by faulty sensory awareness. 'Beware of the printed matter,' said Alexander: 'you may not read it as it is written down.'[2]

The Hands-on-the-Back-of-the-Chair

You can do the procedure seated or standing, in a monkey or lunge. Normally, however, you first learn it sitting down. I describe it so, and I shall discuss variations later and in Chapter 13, 'Combined Procedures'.

Two chairs are needed. The type of chair is relatively unimportant; as Alexander wrote, we need to educate ourselves, not our furniture. Well-co-ordinated people find practical ways of sitting in unergonomic chairs. Nevertheless, we may as well use the best available chairs—high enough for your hips not to be lower than your knees, with a firm seat that does not slope forwards or backwards, and without a rim that would cut into your thighs.

The pupil sits facing the back of a second chair. He sits towards the edge of the chair, on his sitting bones rather than on his thighs. This is a more mobile and dynamic way of sitting. As Heinrich Neuhaus said, 'the best position is that which can be altered with the maximum of ease and speed'. Sitting back in a chair makes it hard to move forwards, backwards, sideways, or up out of the chair. Sitting forwards makes it easier for you to point up along the spine.

1. Having decided to work on her pupil's arms and hands, the Alexander teacher proceeds *not* to work on arms and hands. Instead she endeavours to create in her pupil a state of total co-ordination, in which the relationship between head, neck, and back has priority over all other considerations. The teacher handles the seated pupil and looks for a balance between tension and relaxation, strength and flexibility, mobility and stability. When the pupil is seated, for instance, his back should be firm and upright, the spine not slack, and yet the hip-joints should be perfectly free, allowing the trunk to lean forwards and backwards easily, without any loss of length in the spine. The head, too, should be mobile on top of the spine, yet not floppy. This balance is difficult to achieve, as pupils tend to stiffen their joints trying to make the back stable, and collapse the back trying to free the joints.

2. Once the pupil has attained, with the help of the teacher, a degree of co-ordination between head, neck, and back, the teacher proceeds on to the pupil's shoulders. An average pupil tends to tighten his shoulders, raise them up, contract them in towards each other, and rotate them forwards or backwards. The teacher's work consists in inhibiting, with her hands, these harmful tendencies in her pupil's shoulders, and in cultivating the opposite tendencies, releasing and widening the shoulders. At this point, then, the teacher works on the pupil's shoulders *while constantly referring to his head, neck, and back.*

3. Once the shoulders start releasing and widening, the teacher may continue on to the arms. She moves and stretches each arm in turn, in ways that vary from teacher to teacher and from pupil to pupil. The priority is to free the arms from unneeded tension, all the while ensuring that the neck remains free, the back strong, and the shoulders released. Besides freeing the arms, the teacher points them out, away from the shoulders. (Alexander teachers often move and stretch a body part at the same time, thereby avoiding both the injuries caused by stretching a limb that is not mobile, and the dangers of allowing a limb to become over-relaxed and lose its tonus—a light contraction characteristic of healthy muscle even in repose.)

4. Once the teacher obtains the right conditions in head, neck, back,

shoulders, and arms, she puts the pupil's hands on the back of a chair. This consists of taking each arm in turn, stretching it, pronating it, and bending it at the elbow and wrist (more on this later); while continuing to stretch the arm, stretching the hand and fingers, and bringing them around the back railing of the chair in front of the pupil; and, finally, asking the pupil to take hold of the railing of the chair with his fingers, *all the while ensuring that the pupil is primarily thinking up along his spine, and only secondarily concerning himself with the chair in front of him.* Study the two sets of illustrations of the procedure (Figs. 15a–m and 16a–c) to get an idea of how a teacher goes about it.

The teacher may work silently or not. Verbalizing the different orders as they happen serves many purposes. It clarifies the aims of the procedure; it heightens the pupil's awareness of the different body parts and their working relationship in a whole; it highlights the hierarchy of directions; and it helps the pupil memorize the directions for his future solo flights. The words are a mnemonic guide to the kinaesthetic sensations, and do not take the place of the sensations themselves.

The positions of the arms and hands are much less important than their directions. This means that the teacher and pupil can play with variables such as the distance between the hands, the degree of bending of elbows and wrists, the height of the elbows, and so on, without loss of benefit to the pupil, as long he maintains the right directions.

The *end*, holding the chair with fingertips, is of little importance relative to the *means*, the co-ordinated relationship of head, neck, back, shoulders, arms, elbows, wrists, and hands. Teacher and pupil stick to a well-defined hierarchy of directions, which are executed 'all together, one after the other', and no step in the long sequence is allowed to interfere with the preceding steps. If, for instance, while I work on your shoulder you start to neglect the directions to your head and neck, we must give up on the shoulder for a minute and renew the directions to the head and neck. Similarly, if when holding the chair with your fingers you neglect to keep your shoulders free, we must go *all the way back*, to the co-ordination of head, neck, and back, then to shoulders and arms, then to elbows and wrists, before you can take hold of the chair again.

To touch a chair with your fingers should not cause immobility of the rest of the body. The neck remains free, the head mobile, the spine lengthened. You should be able to move your torso easily forwards and backwards, and in full circles, half-circles, and ellipses, both clock wise and anticlockwise. Indeed, this is how great pianists move at the piano, never losing the integrity of the head-neck-back relationship. Even if the torso does not actually move, it retains complete latent mobility. Further, there is continuous movement *within* the torso: the ribcage never stops to expand and contract with each breath. Before further discussing the use of the arms, I should like to consider a few of the broader characteristics of this procedure.

General Benefits

1. *Giving multiple directions.* In essence this procedure teaches you not a position for your arms, but the ability to give *multiple directions simultaneously, and in their right order of importance.* Besides learning how to use your arms, you learn the discipline of many-layered, all-encompassing thought, which you can bring to all aspects of your life. 'If you find the directions too repetitive,' wrote Patrick Macdonald, 'it means that you have not done your homework, as Alexander did.'[3]

2. *Dealing with right and wrong.* Like the monkey and lunge, this procedure is a minefield of things that can and do go wrong. The beginner pupil is likely to misuse himself in the ways I pointed out earlier in this chapter and in previous chapters. With time the pupil becomes aware of his various misuses and of the end-gaining that causes them, and the procedure becomes an exercise first in correcting misuse, then in preventing it. This process of sensory awareness and inhibition is, in itself, even more valuable than the correct use of the arms that ensues from it. There are two ways in which things go wrong in this procedure. In the first, the pupil's misuse is clearly wrong; soon the pupil himself becomes aware of contracting his neck, slumping his back, tightening his shoulders, and so on, and he is bound to agree that these misuses are plainly wrong. He is wrong, he feels it, he agrees with the teacher's assessment of his wrongdoing. There is, however, a second, and more interesting, way in which things go wrong. When the pupil begins to use his back and arms in a truly right, natural way, this may well *feel wrong to him.* He feels that his back is too tense, the arms and wrists awkwardly bent, his fingers strangely stretched. He may even be in pain, simply because he is not used to the right employment

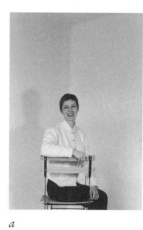

a

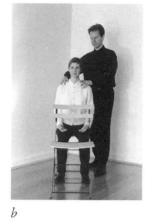

b

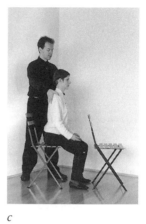

c

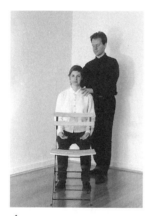

d

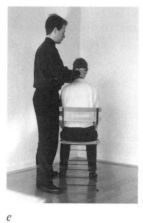

e

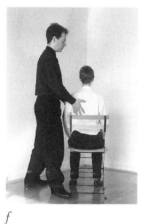

f

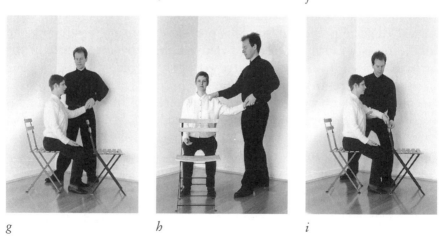

g

h

i

FIG. 15. The hands-on-the-back-of-the-chair in partnership with a teacher

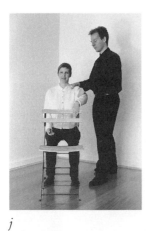

j

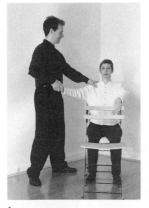

k

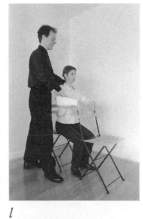

l

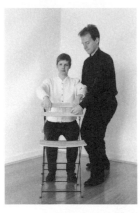

m

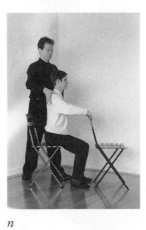

n

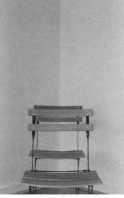

o

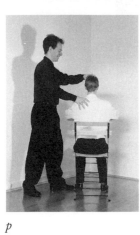

p

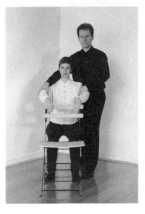

q

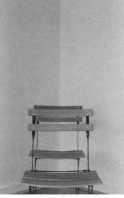

r

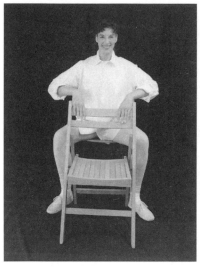

a

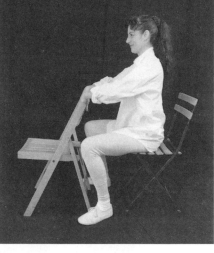

b

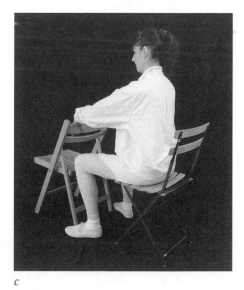

c

FIG. 16. The hands-on-the-back-of-the-chair, solo

of his arms. Even if he is in no pain, the pupil may feel that he has lost control of his arms—a feeling as disturbing and unwelcome as pain itself. Earlier I quoted Alexander on the objective of an Alexander lesson: 'to help you to get able to meet a stimulus that always puts you wrong and to learn to deal with it.'[4] The pupil of our illustration will be right but will feel wrong, and needs to come to terms with his unreliable feelings.

3. *Gauging necessary tension*. The procedure effectively teaches you how to gauge tension to the finest degree. Up to the precise moment when the teacher asks you to take hold of the chair, you are requested to keep your arms completely free from any tension. In order to hold the chair, you then use the minimum necessary tension. The difference between no tension and minimum tension becomes ever smaller as you progress, until you become able to pass from one to the other almost imperceptibly—a priceless ability, and a sensorial joy. You may have had the experience of picking up an empty carton of milk with rather more force than necessary, simply because you assumed that it was full. Your attitude of mind is wrong, the way you use your whole self is wrong, and consequently the way you use your arm as you pick up the carton is wrong. (Without knowing it, most of us use ourselves in this way most of the time.) Alexander's way of working with arms and hands, invaluable as it is for the limbs themselves, has two greater benefits. It makes the use of the limbs subordinate to the co-ordinated use of the whole self, and above all, it clears your mind of preconceived ideas of necessary tension—indeed, of faulty ideas of 'right' and 'wrong'. What could be more useful?

Directing the Arms

To some extent, if the Primary Control is righted much else rights itself, including the use of the arms. Yet there are precise, specific tendencies that you ought to cultivate when working on the arms and hands. Alexander wrote about three distinct ways of using the arms, each of these uses associated with a phase in the evolution of co-ordination. When standing, people whose co-ordination is least developed point their palms forwards, the elbows in towards the body, the thumbs sticking outwards. The average modern man or woman stands with palms turned towards the body, elbows slightly backwards, thumbs forwards. Well-co-ordinated men and women stand with palms turned backwards, elbows slightly bent and pointing outwards, thumbs towards the body.

In other words, co-ordinated people *pronate* their arms. *Webster's Ninth New Collegiate Dictionary* defines pronation as 'a rotation of the hand and forearm so that the palm faces backwards or downwards'. Its contrary is supination. These terms also apply to the whole body. You lie prone on your stomach, and supine on your back.

An *adduction* is a movement of a part towards the body, an *abduction* away from it. I may pronate my left arm, for instance, and then either adduct or abduct my left wrist. If I pronate my arm and adduct my wrist, my elbow points out, away from the ribcage, and my wrist in, away from the elbow and towards my body. Let us refer to this particular co-ordinative direction of the arm as 'elbows out, wrists in'. I shall discuss it further presently.

Together, the pronation of the arms and the adduction of the hands create a particularly dynamic relationship between the different parts of the limb, and between the limbs and the rest of the body. Pronation should be the norm in using the arms, supination an exception. Here we must clarify once again the difference between positions and directions. I may change the position of my arms by pronating or supinating them; within pronation or supination, I may have different directions operative in the arms: contraction, expansion, freedom, tension, limpness, elasticity, rigidity, and so on. In pronation it is easiest to establish the best directions in the arms; once obtained, however, these directions become operative also when the arms are supinated. A violinist supinates his left arm to play the violin. If he learns to direct his arm in pronation first, he will find it easier to maintain the healthy directions in supination subsequently.

When the arms are pronated and the hands adducted, the elbows go out, one away from the other, the wrists in, one towards the other. You can see this relationship at work in the photos of Alexander pupils putting their hands on the back of the chair (Figs. 15*a–r* and 16*a–c*). Study too the pictures of Artur Rubinstein at the piano (Figs. 17 and 18). In both he shows extraordinary use, from the head downwards. His arms are ready for action; they display necessary tension rather than relaxation. Would you agree with me that the older Rubinstein looks even better than the young one? This makes sense; if you use yourself well, you will tend to improve with time, regardless of how well you use yourself to begin with.

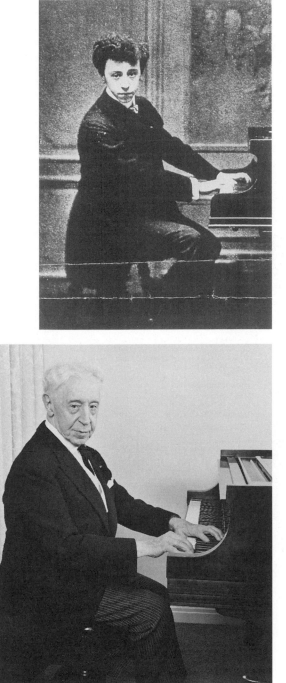

FIG. 17. Artur Rubinstein in Berlin, aged 19

FIG. 18. Artur Rubinstein in New York City, aged 75

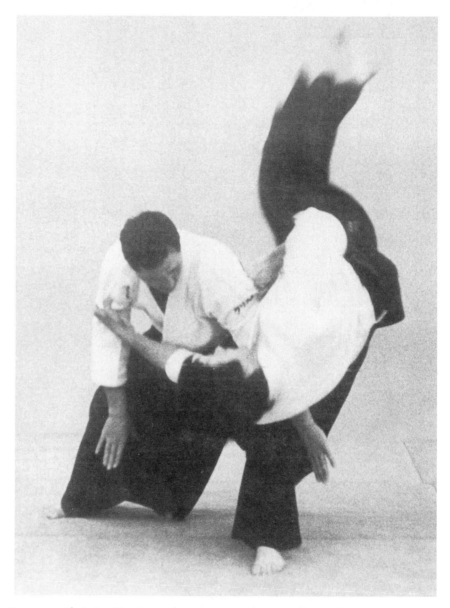

FIG. 19. Christian Tessier with an opponent: pronated arms in action

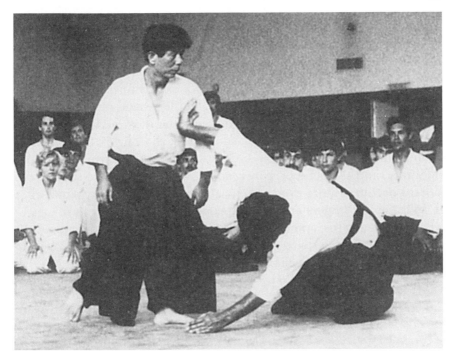

FIG. 20. Seigo Yamaguchi with an opponent: pronated arms in repose

Look again at the pictures of Pablo Casals and Janos Starker (Figs. 2 and 3) in Chapter 2, 'The Primary Control'. You could not find two musicians with more disparate artistic outlooks, yet both pronate their arms and hands at the cello, demonstrating that this co-ordinative relationship is truly natural—applicable to all—and not idiosyncratic.

The pronation of the arms is useful both in movement and in repose. Look at two superbly co-ordinated people, the aikido masters Christian Tessier (Fig. 19) and Seigo Yamaguchi (Fig. 20). As Tessier overcomes an opponent, his arms are pronated, the elbows going out and the wrists going in slightly. As Yamaguchi stands against an opponent, his arms are perfectly pronated even though he is not actively using them. (You may wish to look at his arms as he lunges against Tissier in Fig. 13.)

Their photos, as well as those of Rubinstein, Casals, and Starker, illustrate several principles. The use of the arms must be secondary to the use of the whole body. Well-co-ordinated people *tend* to pronate their arms, although this is not to say that they pronate their arms permanently. Finally, to use your arms well does not mean to leave them relaxed, but to direct them with necessary tension instead. I should like to show the validity of these principles by discussing a few examples of how they work in music-making.

In cello playing the left hand has several separate functions: articulation of notes on the fingerboard, vibrato, extensions between fingers in the same position, shifting positions, and left-hand pizzicato. When the left arm is pronated, the elbow out, and the wrist in, the hand finds itself in the best position to articulate notes; the fingers can extended further and more easily within each position; the left arm shifts more smoothly, and the hand prepares each new position more readily; the vibrato becomes more even and vocal, and easier to control and alter at will; the left fingers are in a better position to pluck the strings in left-hand pizzicatos; and the arm has greater mobility and readiness to move from string to string. William Pleeth writes about the pronation of the left hand on the cello:

The sloped [pronated] position of the left hand has a great bearing on many factors. Because there is a straight line from the hand back to the elbow the hand is centralized, and this not only allows a free and direct transmission of the energy of the hand into the string (giving the sound greater richness and expression) but also enables the hand to create a vibrato which has perfect movement to either side of the point of contact (and hence a core which can be expanded or contracted at will).[5]

The pronation of the cellist's right arm and adduction of his right hand will have a similarly beneficial effect, even though the right arm has completely different functions from the left arm. When the right elbow tends outwards, it is easier to transfer, by means of leverage, the power that comes from the back and legs, through the arm and fingertips, to the point of contact between the bow and the string itself. This is particularly true when playing at the tip of the bow, commonly a source of difficulties in string playing. The arm is also better able to make the adjustments in height necessary to cross from string to string. Pronation makes legato and sostenuto playing easier.

This illustrates the distinction between use and functioning, and their relationship. The same use of the arm—pronated, directed outwards, elbows out, wrists in—affects functioning positively, *regardless of the specific function*: shifting, extending, anticipating, string crossing, sustaining, and so on.

If this holds true—that different functions require all the same use— it should be demonstrably so in instances other than cello playing. Leon Goossens and Edwin Roxburgh write about oboe playing:

Good posture affects all facets of technique. The angle recommended for the instrument will not be particularly effective if the rib cage is constricted by elbows, or stomach muscles cramped by a lazy seating posture. The whole body is active in controlling the presentation of the sound, so that if any part of the trunk evades contribution of poise to the general physical posture faults in the production will arise. Elbows should be poised away from the ribs to allow full expansion when a breath is inhaled.[6]

The elbows-out, wrists-in relationship at the piano is best examined in a video of Artur Rubinstein at the piano. I recommend his 'Last Recital for Israel' (RCA),[7] in which cameras show him in profile, from the front, from the back, and from above. His mastery at the piano is astonishing, and the elbows-out, wrists-in relationship is clearly at work when he plays.

Otto-Werner Müller, a superb musician and arguably today's finest conducting teacher (at the Juilliard School in New York and the Curtis Institute in Philadelphia), has said that the best orchestral sound is obtained when the conductor points his elbows out and his wrists in.[8] This is beautifully illustrated by the picture of the young Leopold Stokowski (Fig. 21). We started our discussion of arms and hands with an experiment where someone lifts his arms in front of himself. Stokowski is doing precisely that; notice how he uses his arms in complete harmony with his head, neck, and back.

Power and Strength in the Arms

The issue of power and muscular strength is a great stumbling-block when changing the use of the arms. Most people associate their mental conception of power with a certain feeling of tension in the muscles of the body. If the feeling is absent, so will be the *perception of power*. In other words, I will believe myself powerless, incapacitated even, unless I can feel the muscular effort I usually exert when using my arms, whether I open jars, play fortissimo chords on the piano, or carry a tuba upstairs.

To play loudly the average pianist lifts his shoulders, pulls his back down, and bears down on the piano keys with contracted arms, wrists, hands, and fingers. As Alexander wrote, he *'believes himself to be merely overcoming what he regards as essential inertia, when he is really fighting the resistance of undue antagonistic muscular action exerted by himself, a resistance of which he is not consciously aware'*.[9] First he creates tensions within himself, then he fights against these

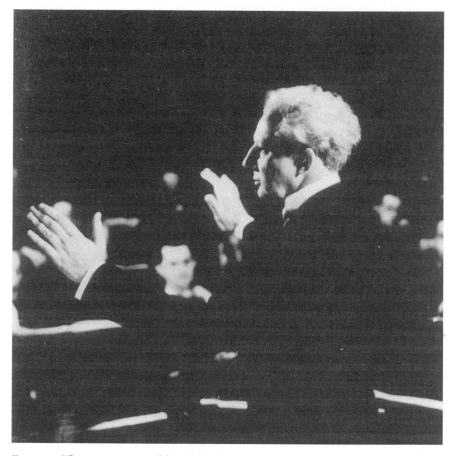

FIG. 21. The young Leopold Stokowski

very tensions, believing all the while that he is merely using the force needed to play loudly. In fact loud playing requires greater relaxation, and less effort, than quiet playing. Gerhard Mantel makes this point in relation to cello playing:

The musculature holding up the arm is relieved of the amount of pressure that rests on the string; the louder the sound the more relaxed the musculature will be.

This rule is easily demonstrated: If the frog of the bow is placed on the string and the arm is completely relaxed, an unnecessary amount of pressure is resting on the string. To diminish this pressure we must use the musculature that holds up the arm. This fact alone shows us how cautious we must be with words like *relaxation*. If one is forced to practice pianissimo for an extended length of time (perhaps because the neighbours are asleep), the arm tires much faster than in loud playing because the muscles must actively hold up the entire arm, including the bow.[10]

The same applies to all situations where the use of the arms is required (piano playing, conducting) and to situations where loudness is not dependent on the use of the arms (singing, playing wind instruments). This is not to say that you should play loudly all the time, only that loud playing is accomplished with less effort and greater confidence and freedom, and should constitute the *norm* of playing. (I shall return to this issue in Chapter 18, 'Norms and Deviations'.)

Yet for this norm to be truly healthy, you must attain it by the right co-ordinative means. The source of physical power, in music-making and otherwise, lies in the back, not the arms. (You do not need the built-up back muscles of an athlete; remember our discussion of swimming in Chapter 1. If the back is well co-ordinated, it will be by definition strong, even in the absence of bulky or taut muscles.) Janos Starker wrote: ' "Relaxed" playing is in reality the even distribution of muscle tension. . . . The [physical] power is aimed at the contact points on the strings, via the bow and the left fingers. The power of the arm originates in the back muscles. . . . When lifting the arms, the back muscles, not those of the upper arm, are required for the necessary power.'[11]

It is difficult to describe what a powerful back and free arms should feel like. Free arms are not limp or lifeless, just as a powerful back is not corpulent or rigid. The muscle tone characteristic of free arms is that of the grip of a baby or infant—lively, firm yet supple. The handshake of an upright, quietly self-assured man or woman gives a similar feeling. When an experienced, caring doctor handles a patient with this kind of touch—secure, warm, reassuring, life-giving—the patient immediately responds by relaxing and opening up. So should a piano when touched by the pianist.

There is a saying attributed variously to Ferruccio Busoni and Dinu Lipatti: 'A pianist should play with arms of spaghetti and fingers of steel.' This somewhat puzzling idea is not inaccurate from Alexander's point of view. Musicians often play with 'shoulders, elbows, and wrists of steel'. If, however, the back becomes the source of power, the arms can become spaghetti-like. H. H. Stuckenschmidt quotes Walter Niemann on the subject of Busoni's playing: 'quite incomprehensible, this modern way of playing octaves, light as a feather, all the strain taken by the back muscles'.[12]

Alexandrian work on arms and hands leads to increased awareness and co-ordination, which have healing effects on bursitis, tennis elbow, tendonitis, carpal tunnel syndrome, and so on. These injuries are caused at least in part when the different joints and other limb parts do work that is intended for the back.

Using a powerful back to free the arms affects every facet of music-making. Changes in the quality of sound are particularly striking. In piano playing, to give a single example, the Alexandrian use of back and arms naturally leads to a kind of sonority that is freely resonant, vocal-like, powerful yet luminous, plastic, compellingly alive. Nobody who has heard Ferruccio Busoni's single surviving recording (of Bach, Beethoven, Chopin, and Liszt)[13] can fail to be touched by his extraordinarily beautiful sound. This was, undoubtedly, a result of his entire personality and musicianship. Yet his sound quality cannot be dissociated from the relationship between his back and arms, a tangible reality that the Alexander Technique does much to address.

I do not suggest that all pianists should sound like Busoni, or like each other. Sound quality is and will always remain personal. Busoni's sound is exclusively his. Yet it shares certain qualities with those of Guiomar Novaes, Magda Tagliaferro, Dinu Lipatti, Clara Haskil, and Vlado Perlemuter. In contrast, the sounds of Glenn Gould belong in a different category. (The reader may well argue that he prefers Gould to Lipatti. Yet it was Gould's feats of rhythmic forward motion which signalled his genius, not his sound-quality.)

Bilateral and Quadrilateral Transfer

So far we have discussed the use of the arms mostly while sitting down. Their directions remain the same when you stand or walk.

At first, to work on the arms while standing or moving may seem harder, because of the many simultaneous directions to consider. In the long term, however, it is nearly impossible to achieve good use of the arms without reference to the legs, because of the phenomenon of *quadrilateral transfer*. The use of the left arm, for instance, always affects the use of the right arm, and vice versa. This we call *bilateral transfer*. It has been studied scientifically, although it is only partially understood:

More than a century ago, Yale researchers found that if you exercised, say, your right index finger, your left one would also get stronger. 'We don't exactly know what causes the muscle growth, but we found that cross-education [training single limbs in alternation] exploits the spinal-cord reflex and leads to faster strength gains than conventional training,' says Joseph Greenspan, M.D., medical director of the Texas Back Institute.[14]

In badly co-ordinated people, bilateral transfer hinders the use of the whole self, as the inadequacies of one limb affect the use of the opposite limb. In well-co-ordinated people, however, bilateral transfer enhances good use, since the strengths of a good limb then tend equally to be reflected in the use of the opposite limb, and the use of both limbs becomes harmonious. Naturally enough, a badly co-ordinated person may use bilateral transfer to *acquire* good co-ordination.

In quadrilateral transfer, the use of any limb affects the use of every other limb. The use of one leg influences the use of the other leg *and* the use of both arms. Some musicians, for instance, contract their feet when playing—often because of the bad habit of keeping time by tapping with the feet. Classical musicians usually tap in irregular, unmetronomic ways; often, they are not aware of the tapping or of its irregularity, or of the attendant misuse of the feet. Their tapping is an effort to make up, externally, for a lack of *internal* rhythmic clarity. If you misuse your feet (by tapping or otherwise), you are bound to activate compensating mechanisms in the legs, then the hips, then the torso, and so on to the upper limbs. (I shall discuss rhythm further in Chapter 16, 'Daily Practice'.)

Most musicians regard their upper and lower limbs as completely different in nature and in functioning, and concentrate on the use of their upper limbs. Like bilateral transfer, however, quadrilateral transfer can be a force for good or for bad. By neglecting the use of their legs and feet, musicians allow quadrilateral transfer to work *against* their total co-ordination, rather than for it.

It is useful to think of yourself as an 'uprighted quadruped', rather than a biped. Playing the violin, conducting, and singing all require the co-ordinated use of all limbs. It is therefore extremely useful to combine the hands-on-the-back-of-the-chair with a monkey, a lunge, or the movement from sitting to standing and vice versa. Please refer to Chapter 13, 'Combined Procedures'.

The directions for the use of the arms are essentially the same whether you are walking, driving a car, or playing the violin. By cultivating these directions at all times, you can improve your music-making even when not practising. Your arms will be readier for playing or conducting if you have been cultivating the right tendencies before you handle an instrument or an orchestra. Pay attention to your arms as you walk, for instance, and quadrilateral transfer will make walking a better use of your time than practising your instrument for hours and hours every day. Even as you ride a bus or lie on your back at home, you may carry on directing your arms. It is good fun to learn to direct your arms at a restaurant, for instance, as you eat with friends. The challenge is to direct without becoming self-conscious, and without giving your friends cause to think that you are an Alexandroid.

The Arms and Singing

Singers may seem concerned with the use of their arms primarily in connection with operatic acting and moving. And yet, because the self always works as a whole, even singers who use their arms relatively little, or not all, cannot achieve vocal freedom without good use of the arms. Using the arms well can and should enhance the use of the rest of the self, including the voice.

When you use your arms well, an interesting phenomenon takes place: *the arms support the back, and the back supports the arms.* (All good dancers attest to this.) The hands-on-the-back-of-the-chair helps you expand your back, free your ribcage, and increase your intra-thoracic capacity and respiratory efficiency. To use the arms well and to breathe well become therefore synonymous. The better a singer uses her arms, the better she will sing. Singers (and all others) may execute the hands-on-the-back-of-the-chair in connection with the whispered 'ah', which I shall discuss in the next chapter.

Accidental Damage to the Hands

Most musicians are extremely concerned with the health of their own arms and hands, as an accident could lead to loss of work or permanent disability. Some musicians refuse to do certain things—opening the lid of a grand piano, lifting suitcases, stripping wallpaper, and so on—in order to avoid both undue contraction of muscles and the possibility of an accident. Reasonable as this may seem, it can lead not to avoiding accidents but to causing them. The more you concentrate on your arms, the less you pay attention to the use of the whole self, thereby increasing the possibility of accidents. Claudio Arrau said: 'I do a lot of things that actually are dangerous for my hands—weeding with a sickle, for instance. I'm not fussy at all. It's important—otherwise you become self-conscious about the action of the hands.'[15]

You always have a choice of different reactions to any given stimulus. Rather than avoiding a situation that habitually makes you afraid of injury or pain, you are better off changing your reaction and losing your fear. Let us look at an extreme example. In the Japanese martial art of aikido, there are a series of wrist locks that are used to paralyse an opponent. If your partner applies a lock to one of your wrists, you may tense up your whole being—in anticipation of pain, perhaps, or simply to try to overcome your partner. Such a response creates the very conditions that favour the presence of pain; the more you resist, the more your wrist hurts. If you let go of the resistance, however, and of the fear of pain, the wrist lock becomes a stretching of the whole arm, and you feel a marvellous sensation of warmth and energy in your wrist and beyond it. Good aikidokas have extremely flexible wrists. Intelligent practice of seemingly dangerous techniques can lead to great overall well-being. Musicians would do well to rid themselves of the anticipation of pain, thereby freeing the use of their arms, wrists, hands, and fingers.

If you do have an accident, the Alexander Technique can then play a role in changing your reaction to the accident itself and in speeding up your recovery from it. Frank Pierce Jones recounts an instructive episode that took place one night after an Alexander lesson:

I was awakened by a thunderstorm and got up to close my window. Forgetting that I was in a country hotel and that the window was not balanced by a counterweight, I loosened the catch, letting the window crash down onto my finger. I had never known how to cope with this kind of pain, but had always been engulfed by the throbbing agony of the sensation. This time, undoubtedly as a consequence of the lesson that morning, I perceived the sensation as a pattern with time-space value and found that I could inhibit the surges of tension that were passing in waves from my neck down my shoulder and arm to my finger. As I sustained the inhibition by keeping the awareness of my head and neck central and my finger peripheral, the sensation changed from ischemic pain to a glowing warmth as blood began to flow back into my finger. In the morning there was nothing to remind me of the episode except a thin red line across the nail.[16]

I do not recommend that a confirmed klutz take heedless risks, but rather that he stop being a klutz. The good use of the self that results from a committed study of the Alexander Technique entails a constant awareness of all things, inside and outside yourself, an awareness that keeps you out of trouble's way. An accident-prone person is a badly co-ordinated end-gainer. If you become well co-ordinated, you need not fear accidents or injuries, to your extremities or otherwise.

Inadequate Fingers

Musicians sometimes blame technical difficulties at their instruments on shortcomings intrinsic to their hands or arms—so-called structural deficiencies. 'My hands are too small,' 'my fingers are too short,' 'my fourth finger is too weak,' 'my joints are too soft,' and so on.

Feelings of weakness in specific fingers are often based on a perception of *relative strength*. My index fingers are much stronger than my little fingers; therefore, I think that my little fingers are weak. What I do not realize is that if I need, for instance, 70 per cent of the strength of my little fingers and 40 per cent of the strength of my index fingers to play the cello, that still leaves me with perfectly adequate fingers all round, even if some feel weaker than others! (I owe this argument to William Pleeth.) This is the 'human design' fallacy, which I addressed in the Introduction. I remind my readers of Heinrich Neuhaus's words: 'The anatomy of the human hand is . . . ideal from the point of view of the pianist and it is a convenient, suitable and intelligent mechanism which provides a wealth of possibilities for extracting the most varied tones out of a piano. And the mechanism of the hand is, of course, in complete harmony with the mechanism of the keyboard.'[17]

Practising localized finger exercises designed to solve a perceived problem easily becomes part of the problem. The great historical example of this folly is the permanent injury that the young Robert Schumann did to his hands while trying to improve the working of his ring fingers. Yet it remains difficult to persuade a musician with tendonitis, for instance, *not* to do wrist exercises, but to work on the use of his self instead, tendonitis being but a symptom of misuse of the whole self. 'Specific prevention is permissible only under conditions of non-doing, not of doing,' Alexander said.[18]

A conscientious musician does not indulge in feelings of anatomical inadequacy. Small hands, short fingers, weak fingers are but flimsy excuses for end-gaining behaviour. Regardless of their size and shape, hands used in harmonious co-ordination with the whole self have all the power, suppleness, precision, and speed needed for every task. To master the use of the arms and hands without harming themselves, all musicians must acquire healthy practising habits, which I shall discuss in Chapter 16, 'Daily Practice'.

11 *The Whispered 'Ah'*

The Whispered 'Ah' Described

The whispered 'ah' takes pride of place among the procedures developed by Alexander. Sir George Trevelyan was on Alexander's first training course for teachers in the 1930s. We read in his diary: 'Asked what he considered the essential way for a sedentary worker to keep in condition, F. M. said without hesitation: "The whispered 'ah', particularly over the chair." '[1]

You can do a whispered 'ah' anywhere and at any time: lying down, sitting, standing, in a monkey or lunge, with your hands on the back of a chair. Because of the difficulties the whispered 'ah' presents to a beginner, however, it is easier first to learn it lying down, in the semi-supine position (on your back, knees bent, feet down; see the next chapter). But keep in mind that it is not in this position that you will get the most out of the whispered 'ah'.

Like all Alexander procedures, the whispered 'ah' is useless, perhaps even harmful, if you do it without thinking up along the spine. If you perform a whispered 'ah' unassisted by an expert in 'thinking up', you risk creating more tensions than you have already. Be warned, then: when I write 'think up', or 'open your mouth', please read 'let your teacher take you up along the spine', 'let your teacher open your mouth for you'.

1. Inhibit your desire to do what you feel to be the right thing. Give up the idea of performing well, or of being in command of the situation, or of pleasing the teacher. Think up along the spine. Let the neck be free, to let the head go forwards and up, to let the back lengthen and widen, all together, one after the other. Allow the never-ending flow of information, from within the self and without, to reach your senses: do not concentrate, do not hypnotize yourself, and carry on watching, listening, and breathing.

2. While thinking up along the spine, smile or grimace, thereby

exposing your upper teeth. It is not necessary to curl the upper lip in a snarl, nor to tighten the muscles of your forehead or around your eyes. The upper lip should move independently of the other facial muscles, and above all independently of the neck: smiling or grimacing should not cause the neck to tighten.

3. While thinking up and smiling, move your lower jaw forwards—in other words, place your lower teeth slightly in front of the upper ones, rather than behind them (where they are normally placed). Moving the lower jaw forwards is difficult for many beginners. To do so while smiling, and without tightening the neck, seems nearly impossible at first, which demonstrates a lack of independence between lips, tongue, jaw, and neck. Some pupils, when trying to move the jaw, move the lower lip instead—that is, they pout. Others open the mouth instead of moving the jaw forwards. It is quite amusing, really. If you are clever, you will enjoy this maddening lack of self-control while it lasts.

4. While thinking up and smiling, and without letting your lower jaw recede, open your mouth. Here most pupils usually move their heads back in space, stiffen their necks, retract their jaws, and lose their smiles. You should be able to open your mouth by dropping your lower jaw away from the upper, rather than by lifting the upper jaw away from the lower. (You should be able equally to move your head back in space without shortening your spine. In other words, you should be able to open your mouth without moving your head and to move the head without shortening your spine.)

5. While thinking up and smiling, and without letting your jaw recede and your mouth close, exhale on a nearly silent, whispered 'ah' vowel. Most pupils will be completely out of breath even before they exhale, proving that they 'concentrate on doing the right thing' to the extent of forgetting to breathe normally. After they realize that they run out of breath before performing the whispered 'ah', they set on the strategy of puffing themselves up like great frogs, in order to have lots of air in reserve for the big moment. They are simply substituting a wrong act for another, as the whispered 'ah' is not a chest-capacity contest, but a procedure to co-ordinate the whole self. When you execute a series of whispered 'ah's well, you need not save up air; you need not take an extra breath at the last minute, before exhaling; *you will always have enough air in your lungs to whisper an 'ah' of some length.* Do not try to control your breath, and it will be perfectly controlled! Another common misuse consists in forcibly squeezing all the

breath out of the lungs. This is achieved by a wilful contraction of the ribcage, during which most pupils shorten their spines, narrow their backs, and contract the neck, shoulders, and arms. Evidently you can and should always perform your whispered 'ah' without forcing or squeezing, regardless of how loudly or quickly you do it.

6. After having exhaled, and while still thinking up, close your mouth without contracting the jaw or snapping the teeth, relax your upper lip, and breathe in through your nose. The cycle of the whispered 'ah' is complete.

You can perform the entire cycle in two seconds or in two minutes, depending on your needs, aims, and abilities. As with all Alexander procedures, each intermediate step is an end in itself. Practise each step on its own, as many times as you wish, before going on to other steps. For instance, you can grimace a few times before you attempt to grimace and move the jaw forwards at the same time; or you can open and close your mouth several times before whispering an 'ah'.

Variations

There are many variations on the whispered 'ah'. In a bid to avoid creating new tensions, some teachers do not insist on the smile or grimace, or moving the jaw forwards. Yet violinists and violists, for instance, often suffer from retracted jaws and should become able to redirect their jaws forwards as needed. Indeed, to have perfect mobility of the jaw is a natural human endowment, and *not* to work on it is not a solution to the problems of a frozen jaw. Although different variations of the whispered 'ah' all have their worth, a well-co-ordinated pupil should be able to do *all variations*, including the most difficult ones. The 'ah' itself can be varied; you can start it with a gentle glottal stroke, which makes the outflow of breath easier to control, or without it, which makes the throat freer.

It is impossible to describe the sound of the whispered 'ah'. Obviously you must keep the throat free and the tongue relaxed, and you must not make any extraneous noises, such as a smoker's clearing of his throat, a hiss, a snarl, a gurgle, or the noises of forceful defecating. Yet the 'ah' should not be completely silent either. The quality of the vowel will play a role in determining the rate at which you spend your breath. Do the following experiment. Sing a single, long note at the high end of your vocal range, on the vowel 'ah'. Now do the same on the vowel 'ay'. Unless you are a fine singer, you will find the second vowel harder to sustain: a normal 'ah' is easier to sing than a normal 'ay'. Use this conclusion—that some vowels are easier to sing than others—to infer that an *ideal* 'ah' is also easier to sustain than a *normal*, average 'ah'. An ideal whispered 'ah' too should be easier to sustain than an average whispered 'ah.'

In one of my favourite variations of the whispered 'ah', I ask the pupil to say a phrase at the end of his exhalation, *before* his next intake of breath. A beginner reacts to this in various ways. Often he thinks, in panic: 'I don't know what to say!' and holds his breath, freezes his neck and limbs, and so on. Needless to say, he misinterprets the purpose of the exercise, which is not to test his ability to extemporize, but simply to encourage him not to expel air from his lungs so forcefully that he is unable to speak at the end of an exhalation. (All the same, we all have the ability to extemporize with ease, and do so every day.) Even when I give a pupil the freedom to say anything he wants to—'Open, Sesame', or 'vanilla chocolate fudge'—he squanders this freedom and misuses his whole self, in an extreme effort of end-gaining.

In this situation the pupil often takes a new breath before speaking, usually through the mouth, with an audible gasp. He has no awareness of breathing in or gasping. He is so intent on the *end* of the exercise—to speak a few words—that he becomes oblivious to the *means* whereby he may achieve it.

After a well-executed whispered 'ah' you should always be able to speak easily, and at considerable length. The ability to do so could be considered a litmus test of the success of whispered 'ah's. I like taking this variation of the whispered 'ah' to challenging extremes, by asking a pupil to speak in a foreign language, for instance, or to alternate, within the same breath, segments of whispered 'ah' and of actual speech.

The whispered 'ah' addresses issues of emotional identification and personal growth. This is clear in the many-faceted reactions that all pupils have to learning the whispered 'ah': fear, panic, hesitation, doubt, overeagerness, displeasure, amusement, sometimes even elation. *It is impossible to dissociate so-called 'body mechanics' from so-called 'mental states'.* A pupil who changes his reactions to learning the whispered 'ah' from one of dread to one of quiet detachment is a pupil who has become a different human being.

I once taught a trumpet player who complained of bad nerves before auditions. He was a highly strung young man, passionate in his beliefs and rather too easily excited. His speech, even when discussing everyday matters, was often so agitated that he could hardly finish his sentences. He had lived in Israel, and I enjoyed doing whispered 'ah's with him and asking him to say a few words of Hebrew at the end of his exhalations. He would become so agitated that he was unable to do anything other than babble—and babble he did with his entire being, from head to toe. He was keen to eliminate his pre-audition jitters, but unfortunately he never made the connection between the way he used himself in everyday speech and his professional woes. He stopped his lessons with me without having mastered the basics of the whispered 'ah'.

General Benefits of the Whispered 'Ah'

1. *Emotional states.* The whispered 'ah' flusters more pupils than any other procedure. Some even refuse to learn it. 'I have ugly teeth,' they say. Or, 'My mother used to tell me to smile, and I hated it.' Or simply, 'I can't.' As I have pointed out, the whispered 'ah' highlights the absolute indivisibility of body and mind. Its greatest benefit, then, is to help the pupil get rid of some unwarranted fears and vulnerabilities. The Alexander teacher is not and should not be a psychologist of the 'Tell-me-about-your-mother' variety. In the case of a pupil who finds the whispered 'ah' difficult, we speak of end-gaining as the cause for misuse of the self, and inhibition and direction as its solution, thereby addressing the pupil's anxieties *indirectly*.

2. *Breathing.* In Chapter 8, 'Breathing', I described the misuses of someone who takes a 'deep breath'. Reread the relevant section, and then ask an unwary friend to take a deep breath. As he breathes in, your friend hollows his back, lifts his shoulders and chest, and pulls his head back and down. As he breathes out, he drops his chest and shoulders, brings his head forwards and down, and slumps. In other words, he becomes a human accordion, folding and unfolding himself with each breath. (As I wrote earlier, the misuses of a 'deep breath' are but the misuses of 'normal breathing', made exaggerated and easier to observe.) By taking the pupil up along his spine with her hands, the Alexander teacher helps the pupil *think up* to breathe out and *think*

up to breathe in, thereby eliminating the accordion effect. Notice that the teacher and pupil work on the pupil's use, not his breathing, which remains an effect, not a cause. Many breathing disorders—asthma is the prime example—are symptoms of misuse of the whole self. By addressing the root cause of the problem, the whispered 'ah' eliminates the problem, rather than suppressing its symptoms.

3. *Facial tension.* Because of the release of tension in jaw, facial muscles, neck, and shoulders, the whispered 'ah' contributes to relief of headaches, migraines, and the discomfort of involuntarily clenched teeth. The whispered 'ah' helps to open and clear up the sinuses, and also causes a change of facial muscle tone. Pupils who frown may then become aware of it and able to inhibit it, and pupils whose faces lack muscle tone may note an improvement in their features. There is also a change in the condition of facial skin, due to the improvement in circulation.

4. *Temporal-mandibular syndrome.* Some orthodontists claim that the misalignment of jaw and temple causes numerous illnesses, including dental, skeletal, and other health problems. Dentists refer to this misalignment and its effects as temporal-mandibular syndrome (TMS). I once had a dentist pupil who was a TMS specialist in London, and he was amazed at the effects of the whispered 'ah' on the co-ordination between jaw and temple. According to him, the whispered 'ah' achieved the same results that he aimed for in his practice, but with greater economy and elegance of means. The whispered 'ah' does not rely on mechanistic, forceful techniques. Rather, it helps you to *let the jaw be free.* To paraphrase Patrick Macdonald, 'to let' is the operative word.

Applications of the Whispered 'Ah'

1. *Speech.* Here is a simple experiment. Say the name 'Peggy Babcock'. Now say it quickly, several times in a row. If your co-ordination is but average, you will find it difficult, if not impossible, to say these two simple words. The harder you try to say them clearly, the more you misuse yourself. Do the experiment with a friend and watch what happens to his head, neck, eyebrows, forehead, shoulders, and arms. Speaking requires the co-ordinated action of lips, tongue, and jaw. Head and neck need not move. The whispered 'ah' is an excellent preparation for speech. By co-ordinating lips, tongue, and jaw

it improves diction and clarity of enunciation. As such it has been useful in treating stammering and other speech difficulties. (Alexander included the case history of a stutterer in *The Use of the Self*, and made other references to it, notably in *Constructive Conscious Control of the Individual*.) Note that the stammerer misuses his whole self. The whispered 'ah' is but one of the many procedures—albeit a precious one—he learns to overcome his disability.

2. *Singing*. Although all benefit from learning the whispered 'ah', singers and public speakers are particularly well served by the freedom of lips, tongue, and jaw that the whispered 'ah' entails. When a singer becomes able to open her mouth without stiffening the jaw or the neck, and without contracting the head into the spine, her enunciation, sound-quality, and legato all improve startlingly.

3. *Wind and brass instrumental techniques*. Many instrumental techniques depend on the independence, or rather the interdependence, of lips, tongue, and jaw. Different instrumentalists have different needs, but these needs are all better served by the perfect co-ordination of lips, tongue, and jaw. Consider the role of the tongue in playing the oboe: 'The conditions required of the tongue in supplying the articulation of the sound are derived from a very relaxed position at the base of the mouth with tip resting under the reed, just touching the curled lower lip. . . . Lightness of tongue follows all other facets of controlled technique in the evasion of tenseness and rigidity.'[2] Consider now the role of lips, tongue, and jaw in a particular area of trombone playing: 'By protruding the lower lip, arching the chin forwards and down, and relaxing the muscular tension within the embouchure it becomes very easy to move into the lower register of the trombone.'[3] The interplay of lips, tongue, and jaw obtains in flute playing as well:

Taffanel and Gaubert decry the use of the jaw to control the airstream. There are two good reasons for not using it; it tends to tense the facial muscles and throat, and it discourages concentration on lip flexibility. Nevertheless, many prominent flutists, Marcel Moyse particularly, do use jaw techniques to supplement lip action. The important point to remember is that the jaw is merely an auxiliary tool; it should not be regarded as a substitute for embouchure control. . . . The reason that Moyse advocates use of the lower jaw to modify [the relationship of the flute to the lips], rather than the lips themselves, is precisely because it leaves the lips free to vibrate and to obtain different colourings.

When the jaw is tightened, or brought back, the air column is directed further down into the embouchure hole. This lowers the pitch and makes the lower register speak better. In contrast, projecting the jaw forward raises the pitch and helps produce high notes more easily. Thus, Moyse suggests, the jaw should be slightly tense for soft passages and quite slack in loud ones, just as the lips should be slightly tighter for softer passages, less for fortes.[4]

Note that different flautists recommend different, perhaps even divergent techniques. Yet, true technical freedom consists not in mastering the 'right' relationship between lip, tongue, jaw, and throat, but in being able to execute, without effort or undesirable side effects, *all* the various techniques advocated by different teachers. A flautist who has acquired the complete independence of jaw that ensues from learning the whispered 'ah' can move her jaw without tensing her face or constricting her neck and throat. She can then use her jaw to control the airstream, *if she so wishes*. The whispered 'ah' co-ordinates the whole self, and it invites you to stop what is wrong before doing what is right. Mastering it, therefore, will allow you to benefit better from the many traditional lip, tongue, and jaw exercises for wind and brass players.

4. *Other instruments.* Musicians whose music-making does not depend on their vocal or facial mechanisms—string players and pianists, for instance—may think at first that the whispered 'ah' has no direct bearing on their craft. It is nearly impossible, however, to have a tight jaw and free shoulders and arms. Therefore, freeing the jaw can have a marked effect on the use of the shoulders, arms, and hands, and on total performance. Bud Winter, a great running coach with a string of sterling world records to his credit, speaks of testing sprinters over short distances: 'If [the sprinter] is any kind of athlete, he'll do [thirty yards with a flying start] in three seconds. Then we talk it over and I tell him to have two things in mind when he runs it again—keeping his hands loose and his jaw loose. Invariably, he takes from one-tenth to two-tenths off his speed.'[5] The same looseness of jaw could help a pianist with his passage-work, a cellist with his left-hand shifts, a conductor with the smoothness of his beats and the nuances of his dynamics.

5. *Pre-concert nerves.* Finally, you can use the whispered 'ah' to control pre-concert nerves to a certain extent. The whispered 'ah' is a total co-ordinative procedure, in which you learn primarily to think up and secondarily to use your facial mechanisms, the two together affecting your breathing indirectly. Keep this in mind, and a series of well-executed whispered 'ah's may take your mind away from the nervousness of the situation, helping you regularize your breathing and your heart rate. To put it otherwise, nervousness is a symptom of misuse of the self, and the whispered 'ah' helps to eliminate the symptom by inhibiting the misuse that causes it. I shall return to this subject in Chapter 23, 'Stage Fright'.

12 *Table Work*

Introduction

Table work is a distinguishing feature of the Alexander Technique. Most teachers use it in most of their lessons, some of them sparingly, some almost to the exclusion of other procedures. But the teacher who does not use the table at all is rare.

It is important to recognize the ways in which table work is similar to other traditional procedures of the Alexander Technique. The object of all Alexander work is for you to meet a stimulus that puts you in the wrong and to learn to deal with it. In the monkey, for instance, this stimulus requires you to consider anew your ideas of balance, movement, position, tension, relaxation, and, above all, direction. In table work, these aspects all come into play, and their hierarchy remains constant: directing, on the table and elsewhere, is more important than moving or positioning yourself.

During a table turn the teacher manipulates different parts of your body in succession and in alternation, with the aim of teaching you how to release and direct each part on its own and in relation to the rest of the body. Every time the teacher touches you, you are faced with a choice of reactions: habitual, which usually consists in your contracting your body where it is being touched and elsewhere as well; or natural, which consists in your releasing a body part without tensing or collapsing other parts. Either reaction entails a whole co-ordinative state, rather than a mere bodily response: in one there is anxiety, eagerness, hesitation, inadequacy, in the other there is freedom, calm, release, control. If you can pass from one state to the other, then you will have learned something invaluable from table work.

This is a pointer both to the worth of table work and to its pitfalls. Most pupils find table work extremely soothing and relaxing; table work alone has won the Alexander Technique countless adepts. To receive a table turn from an experienced teacher *feels* great. Yet the purpose of the Technique is not to make you feel good, but to help you pass from the known to the unknown, the known being wrong and the unknown right. At times, this may not feel good at all! Table work can become a bit of a fix, a pleasant and restorative experience. Worthy as this may be, like all fixes it can detract from the true solutions to a problem and become part of the problem itself.

Alexander referred somewhat dismissively to table work, calling it 'lying down work'. He often let his assistants give his pupils a table turn, preferring to invest his own energies on what he considered more vital aspects of the Technique. This cautionary note notwithstanding, table work has become a well-established feature of almost all Alexander lessons. Teachers may start or finish a lesson with a table turn of varying length. It can be remarkably powerful on its own right; used with intelligence and moderation, it contributes positively to the acquisition of good use of the whole self. And—yes, it does feel great!

The Semi-Supine Position

To receive a table turn from a teacher, or to work by yourself lying down, you need to place yourself in the semi-supine position. Lie on your back, your legs bent, your feet on the table (or on the floor), neither too far from your torso nor too close to it and spread about to shoulder width. Use one or two paperback books to support your head. Pronate your arms; move your elbows out, away from your ribcage, and place them on the table; and let your hands rest on your torso.

Because your habitual misuse exaggerates the natural curve of the spine, you may find your lower back uncomfortably arched when you lie down by yourself. Your teacher will normally stretch your back (without over-straightening the spine) soon after placing you on the table. This all-important stretch of the back is more easily achieved with the teacher's help. There are, however, a few ways in which you can lengthen your own back as a preparation for lying-down work, and your teacher will show them to you, usually in the first or second lesson.

Variations in the semi-supine position are possible: in the placing of the hands along the torso, for instance, in the distance between the feet, and in the distance between the feet and the torso. The height of support for the head depends on the shape of your upper back and neck, the surface you are lying on, and your general co-ordinative state. (In the course of a table turn, your teacher may well change the height of the head support as your back lengthens and widens.) There is some leeway in the height of head support, provided that the head does not drop back and down into the spine, nor forwards into the throat. The neck is a continuation of the spine and belongs with it, not the head.

Lying directly on a hard surface is uncomfortable. Alexander teachers use padded tables of varying softness. At home you will need a carpet or rug, or a thin rubber mattress (like an exercise pad). Some pupils lie in semi-supine position on their beds. This is not recommended, however, if you mean to *work on your use*, the sole exception being work preparatory to sleep. It is only too easy to day-dream, fantasize, or fall asleep if you lie on your bed.

Once you have learned the basics of table work from a teacher, you may use it in a variety of ways. Let us now consider how.

Applications of Table Work

1. *Working on yourself.* Its first application is simply working on your use, by inhibiting and giving directions. These should precede and accompany all other applications of table work; without both, lying on your back will not do you much good. While lying on your back you can challenge yourself in many ways. Try to bend or unbend one of your legs without letting your back be disturbed. (This is much harder than it seems.) Give all your limbs different tasks. See what happens to your whole self when you speak, recite, or sing. Do whispered 'ah's. Use your eyes in different ways and try to become aware of how they affect total co-ordination. One of the hardest things to do when lying down is to stay alert and aware, without drifting into day-dreaming, restlessness, boredom, or sleep. Surely this is why Alexander himself was wary of table work. He wrote that modern man needs a *quickening of the conscious mind*. Lying down on your back may make this harder to attain, and you would do well to remind yourself of the true purposes of Alexander work every time you lie on your back.

2. *Rest and relaxation.* To inhibit and direct in semi-supine position is an effective way of resting and of restoring your energies. Some Alexander teachers refer to table work as 'constructive rest'. If

circumstances allow it, you should lie on your back whenever you are tired or overworked. In Great Britain it has become commonplace for musicians to lie on their backs backstage during a concert interval. It is a more effective way of enduring the rigours of concert life than drinking or smoking. Serious Alexandrians develop the habit of lying on their backs often during daily practice, at the end of a long day's work, to listen to the radio or talk on the phone, in an airport lounge before going on a long-haul flight, and on many other occasions. Keep in mind, however, that for this to be truly useful you have to know how to direct your whole self, otherwise you risk contracting your back and neck or unduly softening your spine even as you lie down and 'do nothing'. 'Doing nothing' in the right way does not entail lassitude or stupor, and you will often get the most rest and restoration by lying on your back for *brief* periods.

3. *Preparation for sleep.* The average person misuses himself badly in sleep. In sleep, as elsewhere, we must distinguish between position and direction. It is possible to sleep in a so-called 'good position'—on your back, for instance—and misuse yourself by contracting the head into the neck, the shoulders into the back, and so on. Nevertheless, it is easier to have a well-directed sleep when lying supine—on your back, your legs straightened or supported by small pillows—and with arms pronated, hands resting on the trunk or hips, than when lying prone on your stomach. Lying on your back and directing before sleep can have remarkable effects in the quality of sleep itself, and in the restfulness it entails. Pupils who claim to find it impossible to sleep on their backs would fall deeply asleep after a short while on an Alexander table if their teachers allowed them to—proof positive that habits of sleep are changeable indeed.

4. *Prevention of fatigue and injury.* When you are tired, the best thing is undoubtedly to rest, and lying in semi-supine position and directing is a fine way of resting. Better still would be *not getting fatigued*. Rather than practising for hours on end and then succumbing to fatigue, take frequent breaks in your practice to lie down for a few moments, and finish your work session *more energized* than when you started it. Lying on your back then becomes preventive rather than restorative. This applies to all activities: practising, studying, reading, doing manual labour, and so on. (I shall discuss the issues of taking breaks without losing continuity in Chapter 16, 'Daily Practice'.) Note, too, that the natural consequence of chronic fatigue is injury and illness. Tiredness is of two kinds: from having worked hard, and from

having worked badly. He who works hard needs to rest, and he who works badly needs to change his working methods. If you get in the habit of carrying on despite tiredness (however this tiredness comes about), you are but courting trouble.

5. *Healing and soothing.* Frank Pierce Jones tells an instructive story about A. R., Alexander's brother and himself a fine teacher of the Technique:

Shortly after the war [A. R.] suffered a severe back injury. He had been riding in Hyde Park one morning when he spotted his wife standing on the sidewalk with their young son. As A. R. sat there talking with them, he took his feet out of the stirrups for a moment just as an automobile roared by. The horse reared up and threw him on the ground, shattering the base of his spine. The doctors told him he could never walk again, and for eighteen months he lay in a darkened room with nothing to do (he could not read) but practise inhibition and directive orders. In the end he was able to prove the doctors wrong by walking, first with two canes and then with one. When I knew him, he used the cane only to steady himself, never coming down on it heavily, and could walk, with a curious swaying motion, for a considerable distance, his trunk very upright and his legs swinging smoothly from the hips.[1]

Doctors often prescribe rest following an injury, an operation, or an illness. In some cases rest seems to be the only available therapy. Yet what made A. R. well was not to lie down and rest for eighteen months, but *to direct, lying down*, for that long. Many of the conditions for which rest is a traditional cure risk being made worse by the very remedy. Directing, however, turns lying down into an effective way of tapping into the organism's self-healing powers.

6. *Mental practice.* You can learn a piece at the instrument or away from it, with or without the music. A good way of working on pieces and technical exercises is by lying on your back and practising mentally. It allows you to conceive of the music you are studying separately from your habits of playing or singing, and to cultivate good use in conjunction with an artistic conception. Walking in the woods, pacing your room, sitting, standing, and being in a monkey or lunge all afford opportunities for practising mentally. Lying down, however, by virtue of its stillness, is particularly useful in disconnecting faulty habits of use from a musical conception. Finally, lying in semi-supine position is useful in memorizing scores, which I discuss as part of Chapter 16, 'Daily Practice', and in dealing with stage fright, to which I shall devote the last chapter of the book.

13 Combined Procedures

Complicatedness and Complexity

Each traditional Alexander procedure works on the co-ordinated use of the whole self, at the same time highlighting the use of specific parts of the body. The monkey and the lunge pay particular attention to the relationship between the back and the legs. The hands-on-the-back-of-the-chair deals with shoulders, arms, wrists, hands, and fingers. The whispered 'ah' addresses the use of the mouth, lips, tongue, jaw, and throat.

There is a natural progression to the procedures. It is futile trying to sort out arms and hands before legs and back are working satisfactorily. If the back is not doing its proper job, supported, as it should always be, by well-organized, active legs, the shoulders will have to overcompensate and work much too hard, and the arms will not be free. Although no fixed rules can be laid down, it is often advantageous to learn the monkey and the lunge before learning the hands-on-the-back-of-the-chair and the whispered 'ah'.

After learning each procedure separately, combine them in twos, threes, and fours, thereby engaging every limb and every muscle group in organized activity. This is an excellent way of learning all aspects of directing: the simultaneity and hierarchy of orders, the balance between orders to do and orders not to do, the needed quickness of attitude, and so on.

Alexandrian co-ordination means not the ability to perform complicated physical feats, but to link thought to action in complex ways. Alexander drew an useful distinction between complexity and complicatedness. Violin playing, for instance, consists of many factors that relate to one another in complex ways. Yet for the well-co-ordinated violinist, playing the violin consists of a single act of the will, and as such it is one and simple. In other words, the arrangement of factors involved in playing the violin is complex; their execution in a unified whole is simple, unless the violinist is badly co-ordinated, in which case playing the violin becomes complicated.

On its own, each step in every Alexander procedure is perfectly simple. Even as the combination of steps into a procedure reaches great complexity, the performance of the procedure itself remains simple for the well-co-ordinated pupil. So should the performance of combined procedures, which may entail dozens of separate steps. A complex movement, being but an aggregation of simple ones, is always easy to analyse, understand, imitate, learn, and perform, while a complicated movement is not. The task of an Alexander pupil is to pass from complicatedness to complexity in the use of his whole self.

Alfred Cortot is credited with saying that playing the piano is either easy or impossible. For his gestures to be one and simple, a musician needs to build his craft from the ground up: starting with single sounds, adding simple scales and arpeggios, continuing on to easy pieces, and further on to complex pieces, these last retaining in their core the simplicity of their building-blocks. To do otherwise is to end-gain. I shall discuss this further in Chapter 18, 'Norms and Deviations'.

Combined Procedures: A Strategy

Back to the procedures, then. The possible combinations are many. Rather than producing a comprehensive list, I prefer to outline a strategy for combining. Take (1) a procedure that deals with the use of the legs and the flexing of their joints, such as the monkey or the lunge; (2) a procedure that deals with the upper limbs, such as hands-on-the-back-of-the-chair; and (3) the whispered 'ah', and combine (1) and (2), (1) and (3), (2) and (3), and (1), (2), and (3).

You may do a monkey and then put your hands on the back of the chair; do a lunge and then a whispered 'ah', either one after the other or in intercalated steps; do a monkey first, then put your hands on the back of the chair, then perform a whispered 'ah', and move in or out of a chair as you carry on whispering 'ah's and directing your arms on the chair.

Why should you go through all of this? First, you cultivate total co-ordination and receive its many benefits. Second, some of these activities closely resemble music-making, and can be used as indirect but powerful aids in acquiring and refining technical skills. The trumpeter who lunges, directs his arms, and whispers an 'ah' is activating all of the mechanisms that he uses in trumpet playing—with the added merit of the hierarchy of orders and the absence of aesthetic judgements that habitually hinder the search for freedom. (I shall discuss this last issue in Chapter 17, 'Aesthetic Judgements'.) Third, combining Alexander procedures is good fun—so, why not?

You may also combine a procedure with music-making itself. A cellist or a pianist can play and do a whispered 'ah' at the same time. A violinist or an oboist can play in a monkey. A singer can lunge, direct her arms, and sing.

When the cellist whispers an 'ah', he releases his jaw, drops his shoulders, widens his back, and becomes better able to negotiate a change of left-hand position. When in a monkey the oboist stops moving haphazardly, becomes better able to project a focused sound, and disciplines his rubato.

Combining Alexander procedures and music-making may seem odd, even silly at times, departing as it does from habitual practice. But unusual demands on a musician's co-ordination can break long-established patterns of faulty behaviour, thereby allowing free, spontaneous movement. When you are asked to do something seemingly unrelated to your immediate concerns—a whispered 'ah' at the cello, for instance—you momentarily lose your control over these very concerns. Since habitual control is often inadequate, losing it is a necessary first step in acquiring true, natural control, a control that is not superimposed over old habits but which arises instead from bypassing or inhibiting old habits.

This strategy is not exclusive to Alexander. Other teachers have explored the potential for change in music-making through changes in habitual co-ordination; witness the success of the Rolland and Suzuki methods. But I believe that the Alexander Technique is unique in its insistence on *non-doing*, the pre-eminence of the Primary Control, the inhibition of habitual responses and the direction of the whole self, the use of the teacher's hands to impart sensorial information, and the passage from the general to the particular in every instance.

Directions: An Example

I close this chapter with a run-through of the directions you need for combining three procedures: the monkey, the hands-on-the-back-of-the-chair, and the whispered 'ah'. This is to show you how formidable (and satisfying) a task it is to direct the whole self in action.

1. Let the neck be free,
2. to let the head go forward and up,
3. to let the back lengthen and widen,
4. to let the knees go forward and away,
5. and to lean the trunk forward from the hip-joints.
6. Let the shoulders spread sideways and apart,
7. to let the extension of the arms continue through the elbows, the wrists, and the fingertips,
8. to bring the arms out and around the back of the chair,
9. to let the fingers take hold of the chair.
10. Smile and let your upper lip off your teeth, your tongue gently resting against the lower teeth,
11. to let the jaw go forward,
12. to open the mouth,
13. to exhale on a whispered vowel 'ah',

ALL TOGETHER, ONE AFTER THE OTHER.

Give your directions not thus: 1; 2; 3; 4 ... but: 1; 1 *and* 2; 1 *and* 2 *and* 3; 1 *and* 2 *and* 3 *and* 4 ... Can you really give direction number 13 without neglecting all previous directions?

14 *Working on Yourself*

Faulty Sensory Awareness

Most musicians spend long years taking classes and private lessons. Their apprenticeship is necessarily arduous, as they have so much to learn. Besides the very magnitude of the task, however, a second factor causes a musician's journey to be particularly drawn out: faulty sensory awareness. Simply put, the musician of average co-ordination does not have a precise idea of what he is doing, and passes much of his time unwittingly acquiring and cultivating bad habits, at the instrument and away from it.

Faulty sensory awareness is such a powerful force that practising on your own may be actually harmful. 'Results are rarely satisfactory if a singer, particularly a beginner, practises a great deal on his own on what he calls "technique",' wrote Husler and Rodd-Marling. 'At first the wrong things will necessarily be practised with the right, so that practising is of value only as long as the good intention is being realized'.[1]

The best way for a musician to tackle this has always been with the help of a teacher, whose first role is that of an objective observer. A radical, if impracticable, solution exists. In the words of the singing teacher Viktor Fuchs:

The old Italian master Tosi wrote, 'If the pupil has defects, especially nasal singing, throaty singing or hearing, he should never sing without his teacher being present.' If he disobeys, a teacher should disclaim responsibility. The great Italian masters of the 17th and 18th centuries were able to keep their students under observation as they usually lived in their master's house.[2]

I do not propose that my readers move in with me. The point is that an Alexander pupil, exactly like a music student, must acknowledge the difficulties of working on his own, and proceed with the greatest circumspection. All the same, there exist effective ways of working on yourself, by yourself.

Observation, Awareness, Imitation, and Exercising

To become aware of your own reactions you have to observe them somehow. At first it is virtually impossible for you to inspect yourself without interfering with what you do. Try listening to your breathing, for instance: you will immediately alter it by the very act of observing it. Further, faulty sensory awareness ensures that most of your observations of yourself will not be true to reality.

It is difficult to be objective about yourself. It is a little easier to be objective about others, although faulty sensory awareness makes this objectivity relative only. Unique as each individual may be, there are forms of misuse that are virtually universal in their manifestations. Once you start noticing how people around you contract their head back and down into the neck, it may be easier for you to suppose that you do the same, even if you cannot quite feel it yet. The first step in learning how to work on yourself, then, is to observe others. Looking at the world around you with Alexandrian eyes is extremely instructive, and pleasurable too.

In the right conditions, imitation is a fine way of working on yourself. A great many caveats apply, however, and they merit their own chapter in Part III. For the moment, I note that the vast majority of people misuse themselves most of the time. To observe others, then, means to observe misuse. Therefore you will need to learn to imitate the *contrary* of what you see. This is an education in what not to do— essentially a negative experience, but beneficial all the same.

Yet if you search carefully you will find admirable instances of good use around you. I draw enormous inspiration from looking at well-co-ordinated children at play, at great athletes and dancers and musicians, at animals both wild and domesticated, at (admittedly rare) anonymous strangers in the streets who seem naturally and unselfconsciously at ease with themselves and with the world. Such models of good use are worth imitating.

The Alexander Technique is not about the 'use of your body', but about your *reactions*. Physical exercise in all its forms—sports, aerobics, stretching, body-building, and so on—is not an adequate substitute for working on yourself.

People who misuse themselves habitually exaggerate their misuse when they exercise. In such cases exercising is clearly harmful. If inhibiting and directing *precede and accompany* an activity, however, the activity becomes synonymous with 'working on yourself'. You may, of course, bring your knowledge of inhibition and direction to bear upon all your activities, including exercise. Only then, and not otherwise, will exercising be of any benefit.

To Do, to Be

Inhibition and direction affect every human activity. Whether consciously or not, well or badly, you are inhibiting and directing at all times. With the help of the Alexander Technique you may acquire a constant awareness of inhibition and direction. Once this happens, the Technique becomes an integral part of your life: not something that you do, but something that you are.

Before you get there, however, there may be an apparent conflict between the carefree ease of good use and the deliberate discipline required to cultivate it. Since the Technique applies to all of your life, it seems contradictory to pick particular moments in the day to 'work on yourself'. Alexander pointed out that 'the idea involved in trying to do better at one time than another is merely a myth, a "dagger of the mind".'[3] The well-co-ordinated person does well at all times. Yet before 'thinking up' becomes an acquired reflex, it is indeed useful to choose certain moments to work consciously on your use. At those times the Technique will be something that you do, not something that you are.

Since individual needs and abilities vary enormously, it would be foolish to prescribe a single regimen to be followed by all pupils. A few general guidelines apply in most cases. It is often better to work on yourself for a short time often, rather than for a long while once a day. It is always better to work on yourself preventively: do not wait until you are tired or in pain before you stop your activities to work on your use. If, however, you do find yourself tired, in pain, or simply in a bad mood, remember that working on your use may mitigate or eliminate all such states. Never give yourself excuses not to work on yourself. Working on yourself is not unlike brushing your teeth. It needs to be cultivated, however grudgingly at first, until it becomes so ingrained that it would feel wrong not to do it.

You can work on yourself at home, at school, during a lunch break, in the interval of a performance, while waiting for a bus, sitting on a park bench, and just about anywhere, any time. Keep in mind that working on yourself does not entail your doing the right thing, but rather your not doing the wrong thing. When Alexander worked on himself, he did not simply perform twelve monkeys in a row. Rather, he gave himself the stimulus to do something; stopped himself from reacting to this stimulus in a habitual and automatic manner; directed the use of his whole self; and then reacted, but not necessarily by doing a monkey!

Ideally you should apply the Alexander procedures reflexly—without the apparent help of the conscious mind, and without stopping the flow of movement to consider its mechanics. Before you can 'be' a monkey in all the situations that require it of you, you need to be able to 'do' good monkeys and lunges for their own sake, without the help of a teacher, and independently from real-life situations.

Strive to be able to perform by yourself all the procedures outlined in this book. Understand their inner logic and the underlying principles that bind the procedures in a cohesive whole. Become able to do them easily, in different speeds, in all sorts of variations, in sequence, in alternation, and in combination. Perform each step of each procedure on its own, and all steps smoothly together. Perform all the procedures as ends in themselves, and as applied to all problems of daily life and music-making.

At the end of his long life, somebody asked Alexander if he ever stopped working on himself. 'I dare not,' he replied. Working on yourself is delightful at times, and arduous, boring, discouraging, and even painful at other times. Its rewards, however, make it well worth your while.

Mirrors, Video Cameras, Tape Recorders

When Alexander first decided to find out how he was using himself when speaking, he set out to work in front of a mirror. Later on he added two other mirrors, so that he could see himself in profile or from the back without having to turn his head. What he saw played an extremely important role in his discoveries.

Many musicians have long used mirrors in their daily practice. More recently, some have been using tape recorders and video cameras.

However, mirrors, cameras, and recorders, useful as they may be, all carry certain dangers.

It is possible to look without seeing, and to hear without listening. Sometimes I place a pupil in front of a mirror and ask him to perform an ordinary gesture, like putting his feet wide apart and close together again. Simple as this may be, if my pupil end-gains he misuses himself, shortens his torso and twists his hips, moves his head sideways or backwards, drags his feet, freezes his breathing, and so on. Then I ask him, 'What did you see as you moved?' Usual answers are, 'Nothing,' 'I don't know,' 'I wasn't looking,' 'I hate my haircut.'

To look and to see you need to be attentive, dispassionate, interested yet disinterested, inquisitive yet accepting, critical yet non-judgemental. Alexander was a man of insight, perseverance, imagination, and humour. Without all these attributes, you risk looking at a mirror or a video, or listening to a tape recording of yourself, without finding out anything about what you are actually doing. Worse, you risk passing judgements—'I like it,' 'I don't like it'—which, as we discussed in Chapter 6, 'Action', hamper the blossoming of objective awareness.

Faulty sensory awareness pervades all of our actions, including watching and listening. The use of visual or aural aids does not guarantee accuracy of perceptions. Only an improvement in the use of the whole self—an improvement which depends in every instance on a change in the relationship between the head, neck, and back—will automatically entail progress in sensory awareness.

Seeking out Challenges

In Chapter 7, 'The Lesson', I quoted Alexander on the basic purpose of a lesson in the Technique: 'You are not here to do exercises, or to learn to do something right, but to get able to meet a stimulus that always puts you wrong and to learn to deal with it.'[4]

Most people try to avoid stressful situations; Alexander exhorts us to react differently to them. To work on yourself is to present yourself willingly with a stimulus that 'puts you wrong'. This happens every time you are under stress, or, more precisely, every time you strain yourself when faced with a stressful situation. Then use your knowledge of inhibition and direction to react otherwise.

You can do this on a specific basis, by practising and performing in exceptional (that is, potentially adverse) circumstances; or on a general basis, by seeking out challenges to your co-ordination. In both cases you will be working on your adaptability. Let us consider each case separately.

Specific Adaptability

Claudio Arrau said of playing on unfamiliar pianos: 'One should be able to adjust on stage, instantaneously. From the first chord, you should know immediately what kind of piano you are playing.'[5] The instrument itself is only one of many variables that a musician has to deal with on stage. A cellist, for instance, may have to consider the instrument itself, the set-up of bridge and sound-post, the strings, the bow, the condition of the bow hair, the rosin, the chair, and the end-pin. Further, he deals with the height and angle of a music stand, the acoustics of the hall, temperature and humidity, the presence of noise, strange odours, the conditions of light. Further still, he deals with matters of dress, hunger, thirst, sleep, interpersonal relationships, and general health and well-being.

To develop your adaptability, practise in non-habitual and un-ideal conditions. What allowed Arrau to get the immediate 'feel' of a new instrument was his thorough mastery. Yet, both as a tool in acquiring this mastery (a long-term goal) and as a compensation for its absence, seize every opportunity to play on different pianos, including instruments inferior to your own. Similarly, you ought to experiment in your practice with every possible variable and circumstance. It is true that you should strive to work and play in the best possible conditions. Nevertheless, you will attain artistic and professional freedom not by putting yourself in ideal conditions, but by responding ideally to all conditions. I reiterate here the basic point of the Alexander Technique: not to avoid an uncomfortable situation, but to change your reaction to it.

When faced with unusual or adverse circumstances—playing on a borrowed cello, playing the oboe with an inferior reed, wearing tight shoes on stage, and so on—musicians misuse themselves, perform inadequately, and blame the inferior reed or tight shoes for their relative failure. But since a great musician always makes an inferior instrument sound good (an observation that applies also to conductors and orchestras), it is clear that we should aim to possess not a great musician's fine instrument, but his ability to make the best of any circumstance. This ability is but a function of the use of the self.

In Chapter 2, 'The Primary Control', we studied total and partial patterns and their interplay. In adverse circumstances we let unusual partial patterns distort the total pattern, thereby causing the organism to malfunction. I play on somebody else's cello; I find it difficult to make it sound like my own instrument; I try to make it conform to my musical and technical wishes by using my arms in ways I am not used to; in the process I neglect the co-ordination of my head, neck, and back; I begin to use my arms ever more inefficiently; my playing worsens. Clearly the solution lies in my paying particular attention to the Primary Control, and letting the heightened efficiency of total co-ordination inform the use of my arms according to the possibilities of the cello I am playing on.

General Adaptability

The principle of purposefully putting yourself in the wrong and learning to deal with it applies to every human endeavour. The better you deal with challenging situations in daily life, the better you deal with them in your musical life. It would be beneficial for you, then, to seek out unusual or adverse conditions on a general basis.

Again here we cannot be prescriptive, as different things put off different people. Perhaps you are afraid of dancing or ice-skating; somebody else might be afraid of speaking in public or handling dogs. The idea is to overcome individual dislikes caused by a habitual reaction that is inadequate to the situation. You need not become a lion-tamer or a fakir; it is enough to come to terms with unwarranted fears, and the misuse they trigger. The Technique is not about keeping your balance, but about losing it and not being disturbed by this loss. To work on yourself is to look willingly and gladly for ways of losing your balance and dealing with it.

Part III
The Applications

15 *Technique*

The Unity of the Self

Whether you are a singer, instrumentalist, or conductor, you have your personal definition of 'technique'. Perhaps you have never articulated it intellectually or verbally, but it certainly affects the way you practise, rehearse, and perform. It might be an interesting experiment for you to think through your current understanding of technique, and state a brief definition of it before reading on.

Many musicians would say that 'technique is the physical means by which one actualizes one's musical conception'. This seems reasonable, yet it makes a false assumption: it implies a separation of body and mind which simply never exists. We return briefly to the words of Sir Charles Sherrington: 'The formal dichotomy of the individual [into "physical" and "mental" sides], . . . which our description practised for the sake of analysis, results in artefacts such as are not in Nature.'[1]

By defining technique as the physical means to actualize a conception, you risk equating the technical work of your daily practice with 'training the body'. Such training is invariably mechanical, repetitive, and devoid of reflection or attentiveness. Take a walk down the corridors of a music college and you will appreciate how prevalent this is.

To attempt to achieve 'technical control' through machine-like means is to end-gain. Musicians who search for control in this manner often achieve neither technical nor musical mastery, and sometimes risk injury to themselves besides.

Fortunately, many musicians have enlightened views about technique. 'Busoni', quotes a biographer, 'writes that a great pianist must first and foremost be a great technician. But, he says, technique does not depend solely on fingers and wrists, strength and persistence. It is seated in the brain.'[2]

Perhaps we can already attempt to redefine technique: it is the *psycho-physical* means of actualizing a musical conception. If you accept this definition you will not think of 'training your body' to acquire or refine technique. You will necessarily train the brain, or, more precisely, the *connections* that exist between brain and muscles via the nerves. Alexander teachers refer to these connections as *directions*.

'Technique', wrote the violin teacher Ivan Galamian, 'is the ability to direct mentally and to execute physically all of the necessary playing movements of left and right hands, arms, and fingers.'[3] To speak of directing mentally and executing physically is perhaps redundant. It would be a contradiction to say of a musician that he is great at executing physically but mediocre at directing mentally. Let us refer to both aspects simply as 'directing', thereby highlighting the integrity of thought and action. Then technique becomes indeed synonymous with directing.

Interdependence and Hierarchy

Galamian speaks of the playing movements of left and right hands, arms, and fingers. He goes further:

However important the individual elements in violin technique, more important still is the understanding of their interdependence in a natural, organic relationship. If, to give an example, the bow is held after one fashion, then the functioning of the fingers, hand, wrist, and arm will fall into a certain organic pattern. If the bow-grip is changed, one must permit all other parts of the hand and arm to find their corresponding organic adjustment and their balance, one with the other.[4]

I should like to expand his argument about interdependence in light of the Alexander Technique.

An eventual change of grip does indeed necessitate the adjustments in fingers, hand, wrist, and arm that Galamian writes about. We must go further, however, and consider the use of the hand or arm in conjunction with the rest of the body, particularly the head, neck, and back. We must also recognize that co-ordination proceeds from the head downwards, or from the centre to the periphery. Ideally, then, the best possible use of head, neck, and back should determine the best bow-grip, and not the other way around.

Galamian was a peerless teacher who produced astounding results in his studio teaching. His book on violin playing is a rich source of inspiration. My aim here is only to steer some of his readers away from the temptation of concentrating on the right bow-grip at the expense of co-ordinating their whole selves from the Primary Control onwards. As we will see later, the very definition of 'technique' depends on this point.

Aspects of a Whole

Technique has often been equated with co-ordination, and co-ordination with the ability to play fast notes. Speed and accuracy may be important aspects of technique, but so are clarity, evenness, intonation, and many others. We hear it said of someone that he has 'great technique' but an ugly sound. This is a patent absurdity. 'Technique', wrote Wilhelm Furtwängler, 'must make free regulation of the rhythm possible, and go beyond this to influence the tone.'[5] Heinrich Neuhaus concurs: 'Work on tone is work on technique and work on technique is work on tone.'[6]

The musician with an ugly sound may have great dexterity, which is but one aspect of technique, but he does not have a great technique. A complete technique implies the ability to play legato and sostenuto, in a wide range of dynamics and articulations, in every imaginable colour.

I presented earlier a definition of technique as 'the physical means by which one actualizes one's musical conception'. I then argued that this implies a separation in the workings of body and mind. Now I wish to argue that it implies equally a separation between technique and music itself—between the 'how' and the 'what' of music-making.

Let us return briefly to an illustration I used in Chapter 4, 'Inhibition'. There I compared two different actions: (1) sitting down in your habitual manner, which is activated by a particular mental command and accompanied by a particular sensorial feedback; and (2) sitting down in an Alexander-directed manner, which is activated by a mental command wholly different in nature from your usual command to sit down, bringing with it entirely new sensations. Let us call the first action 'sitting down', and the second one 'thinking up to bend the knees.'

These are not two different ways of doing the same thing, or two different 'how's for the same 'what'. They are two separate 'what's, each inextricably bound to its own 'how'. 'Means conditions ends, directly,' wrote Patrick Macdonald, 'and . . . ends condition means, indirectly.'[7] *The 'how' determines the 'what', and vice versa.* The same applies to music-making: there is not and there cannot be a separation between technique (the presumed 'how') and music (the presumed 'what').

Heinrich Neuhaus quoted a remark of Nietzsche's about writers: 'To perfect a style is to perfect ideas. Anyone who does not at once agree with this is past salvation.' 'This', commented Neuhaus, 'is the true meaning of technique (style). I often tell my pupils that the word "technique" comes from the Greek word "techne" and that it means art.'[8] 'The objective [the "what"] is already an indication of the means of attaining it [the "how"].'[9]

Wilhelm Furtwängler too took up the connection between technique and art:

Previously technique [was] something positive, because it only ran parallel to what it had to express. Since it has become learnable, something—mind you—which was not the case before, since then it has moved further and further from its meaning. . . . The real problem of our time is therefore how to reconcile it with content. . . . And now it becomes apparent that there is yet another technique of which today's world is no longer aware, which is infinitely more difficult. The difference between these two concepts of technique contains everything of any importance that today's world should and does not know.[10]

The problem of which Furtwängler spoke—that of reconciling technique and content—is a specific instance of the goal of the Alexander Technique, which is to integrate the whole self on a general basis. Technical ability is but one aspect of the way a musician uses himself, technique being 'good' when it reflects the harmonious workings of the self. This is characterized by a clear, vital, dynamic, organic, *unifying* connection between each gesture and its animating thought. In the sphere of musical activity, this unifying connection is the very marriage of technique and musical content of which Furtwängler wrote.

Technique as an Effect of Co-ordination

Technique (good, bad, or indifferent) is a manifestation of the use of the self—an effect of co-ordination, not its cause. This makes it possible to distinguish between technique that is imposed on an organism—the sort of technique Furtwängler called *learnable*—and technique that is nothing other than the natural workings of the organism, implicit to it, inseparable from it. Husler and Rodd-Marling wrote:

A word here about the term 'technique.' To define it is a matter of some difficulty, because it is not easy to decide whether technique applies to singing at all; if it does, where does it end, or where should it end? This may be a pointer: organic being has no capacity for living 'technically'; to impose technical measure upon it invariably signifies the presence of an alien force. Technique, in short, is not a physiological term. . . . The perfect singer (ideally speaking) is one who has succeeded in overcoming all forms of technical usage, he is past the stage of needing its help, he sings with a fully liberated vocal organ, from its inmost nature, with every impulse, urge and drive belonging to it. To create is to bring forth from an existing reality; technique is fabrication.[11]

Husler and Rodd-Marling affirmed that technique *does not exist*, at least not in the common understanding of the word. To use yourself is to possess technique. You need not acquire it, nor superimpose it upon the way you use yourself.

The assertion that technique does not exist is, unfortunately, liable to be misunderstood in lamentable ways. An accomplished pianist turned conductor says that 'if you are able to communicate, if you have something in your soul and mind, you can make music without a great technique'.[12] His argument holds, provided that he use himself perfectly. A conductor's very use is his 'how' of actualizing his musical conception; the 'how' being inseparable from the 'what', the 'something' he may have in his soul and mind cannot exist independently of the way he uses himself.

Technique Redefined

Early on I invited you to define technique in your own understanding. Take a moment to reconsider the question in light of our discussion.

I propose to redefine technique as *applied use of the self*. The use of the self, applied to playing the violin, constitutes 'violin technique'; applied to singing, 'vocal technique'. By now you know a fair amount about the use of the self. I shall recapitulate briefly:

- The self is indivisible, and always works as a unit of body, mind, and spirit.
- Every part of the self plays a role in every single situation, and the use of each part affects the use of the whole.

- Use affects functioning, and to change functioning you must change use.
- Use is governed by the dynamic, ever-changing relationship of head to neck, and of head and neck to back. To integrate yourself you must first prevent the misuse of the Primary Control.
- Such integration—a thought-process and a corresponding, inseparable physical reality—determines an attitude towards life which necessarily includes an artistic outlook.

I shall discuss all these aspects of technique as applied use in the next two chapters. Before we conclude, we need to address two questions. What are the characteristics of 'good technique'? Is it possible to learn to make music without learning 'technique'?

Characteristics of Good Technique

Heinrich Neuhaus writes of a pupil who 'because of technical difficulties or some other reason . . . plays "what comes out" and not what he wants and thinks, or—most important of all—what the composer wants'.[13] This gives us some pointers towards what constitutes good technique.

First and foremost, good technique serves the wishes of the composer and the purposes of music itself. Here Neuhaus leaves implicit a certain artistic outlook, in which the musician effaces himself to better serve music—an extremely important point which I develop in the next chapter.

Second, good technique represents a link between *conception* and *perception*. You conceive of something in your mind's ears; you actualize this conception; you assess the results objectively, to verify if indeed you played what you wanted, how you wanted it. Free technique, then, is synonymous with good use of the self, for it is good use which enables your sensory perceptions to be accurate.

Good technique does not necessarily mean the ability to execute difficult tasks. Rather, it is the ability to do the task at hand well. A child who sings a simple melody perfectly has better technique than a professional opera singer who performs a major role poorly. The child of our example is also a better role model than the experienced but flawed artist. I shall return to this point in Chapter 22, 'Imitation'.

Working on Technique

Friedrich Wieck, Robert Schumann's unwilling father-in-law, once wrote in a letter to Schumann's mother: 'For Robert the greatest difficulty lies in the quiet, cold, well-considered, restrained conquest of technique, as the foundation of piano playing.'[14] Wieck's assessment illustrates nicely a well-established belief of how technique can be acquired. It is a view that, though not incorrect in itself, is often misinterpreted, with dire results. As I said earlier, pursuing technical control for its own sake, by practising in a machine-like, thoughtless manner, does not address the real problem of technique, which is to unite it with content.

Do not give up your daily work on exercises, scales, arpeggios, and études—the mainstay of 'technique'. Rather, infuse every one of your gestures, however simple or complex, with a spark of musicality, so that your technique becomes pregnant with meaning. Instead of pursuing technical control first and then applying to it a veneer of musicality, you ought never to dissociate the disciplined, detailed work on what Wieck called 'a pure, exact, smooth, clear, well-marked, and elegant touch'[15] from the expression of your innate musicality.

To work quietly and calmly, which means to inhibit and to direct, is always to the good. To inhibit, however, is not to empty technique of life. It is possible, and indeed desirable, to heed Wieck's advice of working in a well-considered manner while enhancing a gesture's content, rather than enfeebling it. Scales and arpeggios need not be a-musical. Heinrich Neuhaus wrote: '[Leopold] Godowsky, my incomparable teacher and one of the great virtuoso pianists of the post-[Anton] Rubinstein era once told us in class that he never practised scales (and, of course, that was so). Yet he played them with a brilliance, evenness, speed and beauty of tone which I believe I have never heard excelled.'[16] 'The whole secret of talent and of genius', he also wrote, 'is that in the case of a person so gifted, music lives a full life in his brain before he even touches a keyboard or draws a bow across the string.'[17] I shall discuss this all-important point further in the next two chapters. In subsequent ones I shall suggest practical ways for you to solve technical problems with the help of your good use and your musicianship.

16 *Daily Practice*

Mental Attitude

For a musician, to practise is to solve problems. Yet, as we noted in the previous chapter, musicians often practise mechanically, having grasped neither the true nature of the difficulties at hand nor their ideal solution. 'The problem is never apart from the answer,' wrote Bruce Lee. 'The problem is the answer—understanding the problem dissolves the problem.'[1] Diagnosis, then, is the first requirement of effective practice.

Alexander had a particular understanding of diagnosis and remedy. While he saw that each problem had its own causes and its own solutions, he also remarked that all problems share one fundamental characteristic. They are but symptoms of the misuse of the whole self, and of the faulty sensory awareness associated with it. This observation has profound implications for the objectives (the 'what') and methods (the 'how') of a musician's daily practice. Because the means condition the ends directly, let us have a first look at the methods.

'A person who learns to work to a principle in doing one exercise will have learned to do all exercises,' wrote Alexander, 'but the person who learns just to "do an exercise" will most assuredly have to go on learning to "do exercises" *ad infinitum*.'[2] There are, then, two different ways of performing the same exercise: according to principle, and haphazardly.

Every music teacher is familiar with the pupil who has great difficulty in understanding what is required of him, regardless of the simplicity of the exercise or of the clarity of the teaching. The pupil will not listen calmly to the instructions and will not watch the demonstrations that the teacher offers him. He often interrupts the teacher, carries on playing or singing while the teacher speaks, or watches the wrong part of a teacher's demonstrations. The pupil watches the teacher's left hand intently when he demonstrates a right-hand technique, or the hands and arms when the teacher means him to watch her head and neck. He has preconceived ideas of what his own problems may be and what the solutions entail. Even when he has no preconceived ideas about a specific problem or a specific solution, he thinks—or rather, he feels—that he must 'concentrate' in order to absorb new information. Yet the harder he concentrates, the less he absorbs. Some pupils have veritable little panic attacks when the teacher asks them to perform an exercise, even a familiar one.

Inattentiveness, overeagerness, fear of forgetting, fear of missing out, fear of being wrong, preconceived ideas, hurry, hesitation—as a result of his mental set the pupil ends up performing his exercises wrongly, both during his lessons and, more important still, at home. Musicians of all levels take years and years of lessons, sometimes from a single teacher. Yet they carry on performing all sorts of exercises without deriving anything like the full benefit the exercises have to offer. Indeed, musicians often take an exercise that is potentially beneficial and make it harmful, by dint of the way they practise it. *No exercise is intrinsically healthy; it may become so according to the way it is executed.*

Unhealthy attitudes are not exclusive to beginners. End-gaining is, after all, the most widespread of all habits. Watch a master-class, such as those given by Pablo Casals or Nikita Magaloff and preserved on film, and you will see how obdurate an accomplished professional may be when it comes to learning or practising. So-called advanced students and professionals can be worse than beginners. 'A "beginning" student, from the standpoint of technical advancement,' wrote Cornelius L. Reid, 'is not necessarily one who presents himself for his first lesson. . . . Many vocalists have studied for years, *yet they are still beginners!* Indeed, they are rarely as well off as beginners, because their original faults have often been made worse by having been subjected to mechanistic training methods.'[3] What Reid says of technical advancement applies across the range of human activity. Alexander wrote, 'The very essence of change demands coming into contact with the unknown, . . . therefore, [pupils'] past experiences (the known) will not help but rather impede them.'[4] 'People that haven't any fish to fry, they see it all right,'[5] he said elsewhere. Advanced students and professionals have much too much fish to fry!

Good teachers do their utmost to remove all the barriers that a pupil may have created to the correct execution of every exercise. In this sense every music teacher has to be a psychologist as well. Patience, humour, imagination, and cunning are all as important to a good teacher as technical knowledge. We are ready to state the first step in working to principle. 'When . . . we are seeking to give a patient conscious control,' wrote Alexander, 'the consideration of mental attitude must precede the performance of the act prescribed. The act performed is of less consequence than the manner of the performance.'[6]

Exercises and the Use of the Self

Let us now assume that the pupil is ready to perform the exercise to principle. Besides an open mind and a calm attitude, principle requires that *every exercise, without exception, be executed in a context of total co-ordination.* 'All exercises are fundamentally the same', wrote Alexander, 'in the sense that the activity which goes to their performance is inseparable from the habitual manner of general use of the performer.'[7]

Directing the whole self, then, should precede and accompany the execution of every exercise. I give a cello pupil an exercise for left-hand articulation. I insist on (1) a clear mental attitude, free from fear or preconceived ideas; (2) the concerted use of head, neck, back, shoulders, arms, legs, and feet, with particular attention paid to preventing the misuse of the Primary Control; (3) the pupil's ability to watch, listen, breathe, and speak during the execution of the exercise, thereby ensuring that he is not 'concentrating' wrongly; and (4) the correct use of the left hand as prescribed by the exercise. To heighten total co-ordination, I may also require that the pupil use his right hand when exercising his left hand and vice versa, thereby bringing bilateral transfer into play.

Rhythmic discipline and the driving force of forward motion are further requirements of a musician's total co-ordination. Therefore, every exercise should be performed *rhythmically.* I shall discuss this presently.

Laborious as it may seem, this demanding way of practising ensures that the performing of every exercise is truly beneficial. By working to principle you will not harm either the mechanism you are exercising or other mechanisms elsewhere in the organism. I wrote about Robert Schumann and the permanent injury he did to his hands while trying to improve their use. If you practise every exercise, however localized, with attention to the use of the whole self, you will avoid such impairment.

Working to principle means developing certain constants of clear thinking and good use which, once established, are carried over into every activity. Learn the monkey to principle, for instance, and the lunge and the whispered 'ah' will be easier to learn. So will be playing, singing, or conducting. 'If you apply the principle to the carrying out of one evolution, you have learned the lot,'[8] said Alexander.

About Rhythm

Alexander did not write specifically about rhythm, but Patrick Macdonald wrote of Alexander's discovery 'of the natural rhythm within the human body which exists in the sensory and motivating mechanisms' and which 'has become distorted in most people', thereby contributing to 'the ill-health and distress of many so-called mental and physical diseases'.[9] Breathing, circulation, love-making, locomotion all demonstrate that healthy functioning is naturally rhythmic.

Good rhythm improves use and functioning, at the same time that good use improves rhythm: they feed each other. Jerky, irregular, accented movements are never free; rhythmic discipline is the first requirement for a musician in search of freedom. 'The musician's bible', said the great conductor Hans von Bülow, 'begins with the words: "In the beginning there was rhythm."'[10]

When I speak of rhythmic discipline I am not referring exclusively to the precision of a metronome. Precision is indeed essential to good rhythm, and I maintain that the metronome is a musician's best friend. Playing to a metronome, however, is similar to looking at yourself in a mirror. The mirror shows you what you look like, but in itself it cannot make you beautiful. Make a change in your posture, for instance, and with the aid of the mirror you may see the difference. The metronome will not make you precise, but by listening carefully to it you can tell whether your rhythm is precise or not.

Perfect rhythm includes precision, but also energy, dynamism, impetus—what musicians usually call *forward motion*. This is nearly indescribable. Forward motion is part of the quality in music that makes you want to tap your foot or pretend you are the conductor. Speaking of the rhythmic element in Sviatoslav Richter's playing, Heinrich Neuhaus quoted Goethe: 'You think that you push but you are being pushed.'[11] Forward motion makes music compelling, and it adds a liveliness to rhythmic discipline that is lacking in mere metronomic precision.

Many musicians distort the rhythm of a musical phrase or exercise in order to accommodate a technical ineptness. A musician who is

learning a new piece may rush over easy passages and slow down difficult ones. He may claim he is 'concentrating' on sound-production,
or fingering, or getting the notes, and so on, and therefore 'the rhythm
is not important'. Yet virtually all difficulties are conquered *through*
good rhythm, not before it, and above all not separate from it. Good
rhythm is the means whereby a musician may acquire freedom, and
for him to neglect it is to end-gain.

The simplest exercise and the most complex passage should always
be executed rhythmically. Husler and Rodd-Marling wrote:

> By rousing a muscle's rhythmic sense, deep-seated energies within it are released
> (as in all forms of organic life, muscles are rhythmically constituted). This makes
> for ease and freedom of movement. Life without rhythmic content is never very
> vital. A muscle that works unrhythmically is always a hampered one, and to prac-
> tise unrhythmically means that in time every muscle is certain to deteriorate. As
> Plato defined it, 'rhythm regulates movement.'[12]

You have several choices when you cannot play a difficult passage up
to tempo: play at a slower tempo, simplify the passage, or slow down
the rate of changes of variables without changing the tempo (I shall
explain this last choice in Chapter 20, 'Variables and Constants'). In
every case you ought to play the passage with perfect rhythm; otherwise you will not be able to regulate the body movements you need
to master the difficulty in the passage.

Husler and Rodd-Marling addressed the relationship between
rhythm, functional freedom, and musicality. A fully healthy vocal organ,
they wrote, 'is charged with rhythm so that it possesses both speed and
flexibility. Unless the singer happens to be miraculously untalented,
phrasing of a simple kind ensues automatically, as a result of the correct physical-physiological movements in the vocal organ. What is
more, its good condition stimulates the singer's inventiveness.'[13]

In other words, good use is intrinsically rhythmic, and contains in
itself the very seeds of musicality. This is an extremely important point,
which I made in the previous chapter, 'Technique', and to which I shall
return in the next one, 'Aesthetic Judgements'.

Working on Rhythm Away from the Instrument

By the way he moves as he plays, sings, or conducts, a musician often betrays inadequacies of rhythmic control. While playing a

series of syncopations, for instance, some musicians bob up and down, shortening their bodies in the process, or breathe in noisily through their noses to signal the beats to which the music syncopates. Another common manifestation of rhythmic inadequacy is trying to keep time or count beats by tapping with the feet or nodding. Such gestures do not express rhythmic vitality; rather, they compensate for the lack of inner rhythm. Like all compensatory mechanisms, they end up contributing to the problem for which they are presented earnestly as a solution.

I propose two strategies to improve your rhythm through changes in the way you use yourself. The first concerns the ability to read rhythms out loud, it requires a clear understanding of the distinctions between pulse, metre, and rhythm and the way they relate to each other in a clearly defined hierarchy. The second strategy concerns rhythmic continuity and precision at your instrument, and it relies on subdivision of pulse and anticipation of rhythmic changes to a melodic line.

Let us consider rhythm away from your instrument first. Think up and place yourself in a close-footed lunge. Keep in mind at all times that thinking up is an attitude as much as a co-ordinative state. Carry on thinking up, and snap the fingers of your right hand in a steady beat of moderate speed. This is your rendition of pulse or beat: a regular division of time. (Musicologists have failed to come up with unequivocal definitions of rhythm and related terms; my own definitions are meant for practical, not philosophical, purposes.) Now carry on thinking up and snapping your fingers, and use your right arm to indicate metre: a regrouping of beats. If your chosen metre is quadruple (four crotchets or quarter-notes to a bar), then your arm goes down, to the left, to the right, up, and down again. Carry on thinking up, snapping your fingers, and moving your right arm, and use your voice to say a rhythm out loud: a combination of subdivisions and regroupings of pulse. To read rhythms out loud, use syllables that you find easy to pronounce and enunciate (for instance, 'tam', 'taddam', and so on).

Simple as this may seem, it is a laboratory of things that can go wrong. How steady is your beat? What happens to your wrist and arm when you snap your fingers? What happens to your head, neck, and back when you move your right arm? Do you move your arm heavily or lightly, timidly or confidently? Do you stiffen your left arm? Are you able to keep a continuous pulse as you speak? When you speak do you move your head about? What happens if you try to read a complex rhythm?

In this exercise you are being asked to do many things, all together, one after the other, in a definite hierarchy. Think up; snap your fingers (pulse); wave your arm (metre); use your voice (rhythm). The rhythm is the end to be achieved; thinking up and producing clear pulse and metre are the means whereby the end may be achieved. By concentrating on the end, you are only too likely to neglect the means; the end suffers as a result. You may wish to perform this exercise with a friend; by observing somebody else's struggles, you may learn a great deal about your own difficulties and misuses.

Cultivate the ability to think up in everything you do. Then cultivate the ability to keep a rock-solid pulse going at the same time you speak or move. (When practising with a friend you can do all kinds of tricks to tempt each other to end-gain and neglect the pulse.) Then cultivate the ability to keep both pulse and metre as you speak and move. With practice you will become ever more able to *feel* rhythm and hear it with your mind's ears. Then you can play, sing, or conduct with rhythmic precision and forward motion without misusing your head, neck, shoulders, back, legs, and feet.

In Ex. 16.1 I have set out the different phases of this exercise. Keep in mind that every phase can be infinitely varied; what I wrote down is but a possibility. You will see that the example ends with a passage from the cello literature. It contains both complex rhythms and technical difficulties, particularly of the left hand. By mastering the rhythms separately from his playing, according to the principles I outlined, the cellist will surely become better able to overcome the passage's technical difficulties without neglecting or distorting its rhythms in the process. Indeed, his rhythmic clarity will mitigate, if not eliminate, several of these difficulties.

Working on Rhythm at the Instrument

The second strategy I propose for your work on rhythm requires that you play and speak at the same time. Singers and brass and woodwind players can learn it at the piano. After you understand the basics of the exercise you will not need to speak at all; you can then perform the exercise even as you sing or play the oboe.

Ex. 16.1

a Think up in silence, and place yourself in a close-footed lunge, right foot slightly forwards and outwards, right knee slightly bent, left leg straight.

b Add a beat by snapping the fingers of your right hand.

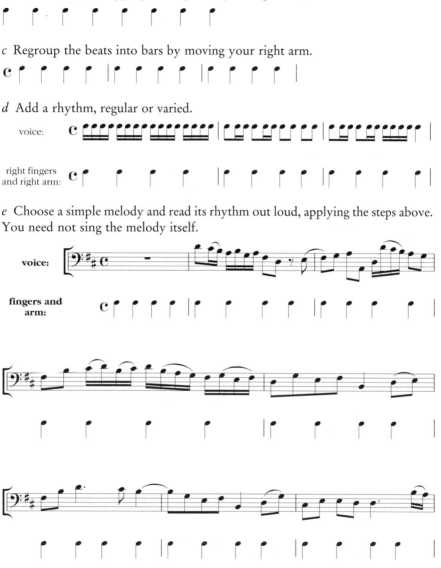

c Regroup the beats into bars by moving your right arm.

d Add a rhythm, regular or varied.

voice:

right fingers and right arm:

e Choose a simple melody and read its rhythm out loud, applying the steps above. You need not sing the melody itself.

voice:

fingers and arm:

From Domenico Gabrielli, 'Canon a due violoncelli'

f See if you can read the excerpt below without neglecting the upward thought, the pulse, or the metre of the passage. You may subdivide the beat and snap your fingers twice for each beat, without changing the basic **C** gesture (down, left, right, up).

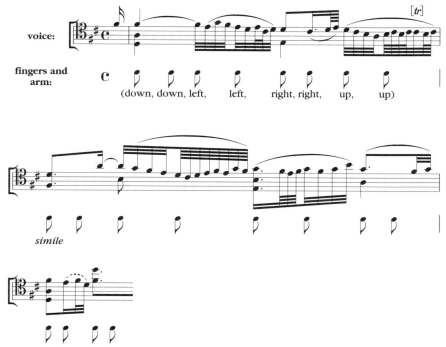

From J. S. Bach, Suite in D major for unaccompanied cello, BVW 1012, Allemande

I wrote earlier of the ways in which musicians misuse themselves to compensate for a lack of rhythmic clarity or vitality. In any given line of music there will be several points where such misuse becomes more likely. These include long notes, dotted notes, tied notes, long notes that come before or after a group of short notes, and others still. In the case of a long note—over several beats, or over a single beat in a very slow tempo—a musician tends to misuse himself as he counts the value of the note with his head, neck, arms, of feet. It would be better for him to *feel* the value of the note, or to measure it *mentally*, with his mind's ears, rather than acting the measuring out with his body, as so doing distorts his technique, his sound-production, and the very rhythm it is intended to help. The same applies to the other instances of rhythmic difficulties. Here is the strategy. Again keep in mind that the variations are only limited by your own imagination. The procedure is set out in full in Ex. 16.2.

Play a long, slow scale. Play it again, and now say out loud those beats in each long note that follow the first beat of the note. Use an easy syllable such as 'tam', or 'pam', with a clear first consonant, a sustained vowel, and a round, soft 'm' to close it. The quality of these syllables will inflect your play; make them convincing, confident but not loud; use crescendos and diminuendos; try different emphases— on the second and forth beats, for instance, on the third beat only. Pretend that you are on stage, and both your playing and your speaking must carry a musical message across.

Now play scales at other speeds and rhythms, and use your voice to say out loud inner beats and subdivisions of beats. Do not say every single beat out loud; let there be an interchange between your playing some beats and saying others. This will make the rhythmic component of your music-making both precise and dynamic.

Ex. 16.2

a Prepare your work by thinking up in silence.

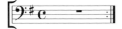

b Play a simple scale at a moderate speed.

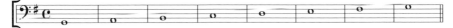

c Play the same scale, saying-out loud the beats that follow the downbeat.

d Make the scale slightly faster and rhythmically more elaborate.

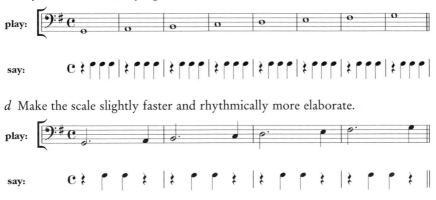

e Choose a different time signature and speed.

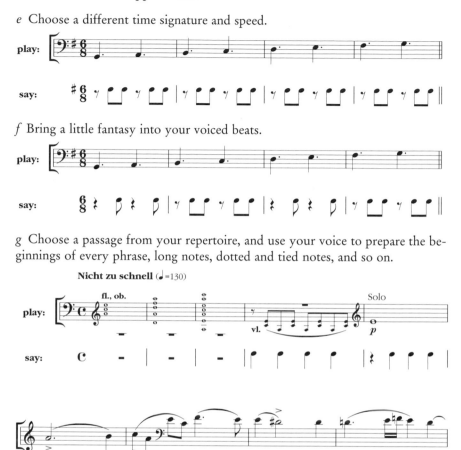

f Bring a little fantasy into your voiced beats.

g Choose a passage from your repertoire, and use your voice to prepare the beginnings of every phrase, long notes, dotted and tied notes, and so on.

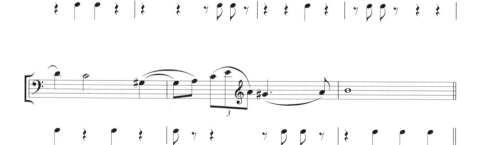

From R. Schumann, Concerto in A minor for cello and orchestra, Op. 129

h Go on to more challenging rhythms. Are you still thinking up?

i Play your scales and passages again, this time thinking the inner beats rather than saying them out loud or acting them out with your head, neck, shoulders, and so on.

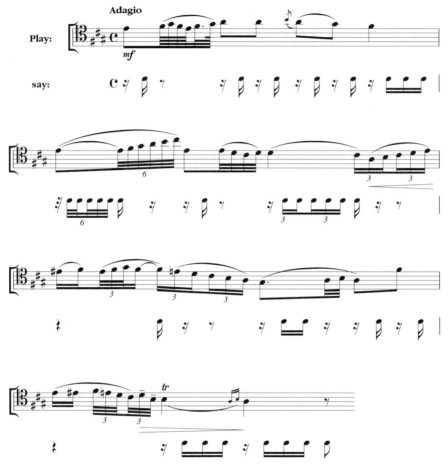

From Luigi Boccherini, Sonata in A major for cello and piano, first movement

Now take a passage from the literature for your instrument. As you play it, use your voice to give metronomic precision to long notes, dotted notes, and tied notes. Let your voice contribute to your ability to play legato and sostenuto. Use it too as you prepare the changes from long notes to shorter ones. Be as good as a metronome and better than one—unlike the metronome, you are imaginative and lively. Use the voiced subdivisions to gauge your rubato, making it both disciplined and free.

Again it may be useful to practise with a partner. You will quickly see that you (and your partner) normally attempt to create rhythmic precision by misusing your face, head, neck, and various parts of the body. See if you can become able to think up, play, and speak at the same time; do not sacrifice your upward thought at any time. Speak by using your lips, tongue, jaw, and vocal mechanisms *only*, and not your head and neck. If you work to principle you will eventually be able to let your mind's ears take the role taken by your voice. Then you can have all the rhythmic precision and forward motion you need without a single bodily manifestation, other than those needed by the techniques of your instrument.

Before you have achieved inner mastery of rhythm, your gestures at the instrument are primarily manifestations of technical shortcomings. Once you achieve mastery, your gestures are primarily manifestations of your interpretative freedom. I shall discuss this issue further in the next chapter.

Repetition: Right and Wrong

Repetition—of exercises, phrases, sections, movements—plays an important role in daily practice. About repetition there is a simple truth: to repeat something that is wrong is, but for three exceptions, necessarily bad; to repeat something that is right may possibly, but not necessarily, be good. In either case you must treat repetition in your daily practice with the utmost circumspection.

You can justify repeating something that you know is wrong only if by doing so you heighten your awareness of what you are actually doing. You play the cello for me, and I notice that you lift and contract your right elbow every time you play a certain bow-stroke. Perhaps you have never noticed that you misuse yourself in this way.

I may ask you to do it again and bring your attention to the misuse—as a first step in your eliminating it. Here repetition of something that is wrong is useful and even necessary.

Doing something wrong on purpose may also help you cultivate an appreciation of what is right. After you become able to release your right arm in the correct way, I ask you again to do the wrong thing and then contrast it with the right thing, which becomes clearer and easier to remember and re-create as a result.

Now let us imagine a different situation. You are afraid of doing the wrong thing (missing out a note, botching the climax of a phrase, playing too loudly), and the very fear of being wrong causes you to misuse yourself and go wrong as a result. I may ask you to do the wrong thing *on purpose*, which may well help you get rid of the paralysing fear of going wrong, and of the misuse that fear engenders.

Yet these three pedagogical situations are clearly exceptional. Normally there is no good reason for you to practise something wrong repeatedly and willingly. To do so is simply to cultivate bad habits. 'One would suppose that repeated experience of failure would of itself lead [one] to set to work on a different principle,' Alexander remarked wryly.[14] Patrick Macdonald wrote, 'When at first you don't succeed, never try again, at least not in the same way,'[15] thereby reinventing the famous saying.

The pianist André Benoist, who performed with Heifetz, recounts an interesting tale which illustrates neatly the value of not practising wrong things. As a small child, Heifetz was first taught by his father, who also supervised his daily practice. Heifetz, writes Benoist,

was never allowed to play one note out of tune. He was never allowed to hold or use his bow, even for a fraction of second, in the wrong way. When his practice time was over, the violin and bow were immediately taken away from the child and locked out of his reach. The consequences were, of course, that he never had an opportunity to undo any benefits he had gained from his practice time. The upshot also was that he never took a step backwards; and each step being steadily forward, he progressed by leaps and bounds, and by the time he was nine years old (having started at three), he was a finished virtuoso.[16]

The argument for not repeating something that is right may appear less compelling. But 'a human being becomes less human with identical repetition of the same action,' wrote Hiroide Ogawa, basketball coach and Zen teacher. 'Practise [*sic*] shooting from the same spot over and over again is no more useful than tightening identical screws from eight in the morning until four. A different stance. A different position. A different ball. A different player. Now it counts!'[17]

Since most gestures and sounds are usually imperfect, you should attempt to make each gesture different in some way from the preceding one. If you feel the need to execute the same gesture repeatedly, make sure that you vary it constantly and imaginatively. Endless variations, big and small—of rhythm, speed, accent, intensity, tonality, and so on—are possible on each exercise. These alter the outer form without distracting you from the object of the exercise.

Sometimes you may make a healthy, natural, satisfying, intrinsically *right* gesture. To do something right creates its own problems, above all the temptation for you to seek to reproduce the sensations that this healthy gesture gave you. This is a 'dagger of the mind', in Alexander's mystifying but evocative words. You should seek *never* to reproduce the sensations of a right action, but rather its co-ordinative processes, the sensations being but an effect of these processes. 'The experience you want is in the process of getting it,' said Alexander. 'If you have something, give it up. Getting it, not having it, is what you want.'[18]

Reliability and Control

The reason for repeating a passage many times over is that it creates a kinaesthetic memory of the passage, so that a command from your brain will retrieve this memory with ease and reliability during performance. In the hands of an end-gainer, however, both this reasonable goal (to develop a reliable muscular memory) and the method of achieving it (daily repetition) can create obstacles to technical and musical freedom.

About the goal first. Clarity, precision, and reliability are all desirable components of a musician's technique. Yet the musician who strives to achieve machine-like accuracy goes against the very nature of music-making. Wilhelm Furtwängler wrote:

Nothing can be said against precision, but it practically eliminates the most important thing about playing, the intuition of the moment. . . . The possibility of rehearsing *ad infinitum*, which is sometimes portrayed as a special privilege, necessarily diminishes the sensitivity and consequently the quality of the conductor's technique . . . , as well as the psychological sensitivity of the orchestra, which becomes used to typical, uninspired, craftsmanlike work. . . . Improvisation is lost

as both essence and idea. Improvisation, which does not represent a mere accident, an attribute which one may or may not have, but rather simply the source
of all great, creative, necessary playing.[19]

What Furtwängler said of over-rehearsing is, naturally, true of over-
practising and of over-repeating an exercise. Here it may be useful to
make a distinction between *being* secure and *feeling* secure. Just as
most people feel sated only after overeating, so you may feel technically secure only after over-practising. It is a misleading feeling, an instance of faulty sensory awareness. True control often feels like a lack
of control. By addressing this issue on a general basis, regarding your
whole co-ordination, the Alexander teacher helps you to deal with it
on a particular basis, regarding your music-making.

There are musicians who practise the same passage dozens, nay,
hundreds of times. Even if the goal of machine-like reliability were desirable or achievable, would obsessive practising be necessary? Alexander clearly did not think so:

Just as a cat by sheer instinct, the first time she essays to jump, gauges her powers
and the distances with accuracy, so, with more reason and greater ease, the human
subject, by employing consciously controlled intellect and kindred experience in
place of instinct, should be able to direct his powers to a definite ordained end
with less physical strain and less frequent physical repetition, i.e. 'Practice.'[20]

Repeating the same passage unreasonably reflects an intemperate
thirst for control—an interesting demonstration of the connection between ends and means. You will master every difficulty after the fewest
tries if you practise intelligently and economically. Three questions
then arise: How long should a practising session last? When should
you stop? How should you apportion your time during practice?

I consider the first two questions in the next section. To the third
no answer can be given to cover every musician's needs, but you will
find some pointers and guidelines in the sections 'The Objectives of
Daily Practice' and 'Alternation, Continuity, and Endurance'.

The Length of Practising Sessions

It is a truism of musical pedagogy that practising too much is
as harmful as not practising enough. Yet there still are many musicians
of all levels who are bent, so to speak, on practising nearly incessantly,

sometimes clocking eight or more hours of daily practice. Let us restate the case for shortened practising sessions. Theodor Leschetizky was one of the great piano teachers of the late nineteenth century; Paderewski and Schnabel were but two of his many outstanding pupils. About his teaching, Harold C. Schonberg writes:

Among his strictures was the falsity of the concept that long hours of practise were beneficial. He would not think of a student working six, seven, eight hours a day. 'No one can do that without being mechanical, and that's just what I'm not interested in. Two hours, or three at most, is all anyone should require if he will only listen to what he is playing and criticize every note.'[21]

The secret of Leschetizky's teaching, if there is any secret, was his ability to make his students hear themselves and the tone they produced (something in which very few teachers have ever been successful).[22]

It is virtually impossible for a musician, however brilliant, to hear himself with due attention over too long a period of time. This is an indisputable fact of daily practice. 'Don't forget, when a certain amount of effort is expended in practice, like in everything else, you then have to relax,' said Jascha Heifetz, the paragon of violinists. 'I do not think I could ever have made any progress if I had practised six hours a day. . . . Even though I may practise three hours a day it is certainly not three hours consecutively, but rather three hours with frequent intervals for relaxation in between.'[23]

You may argue that it is all very well for Heifetz to practise only a few hours a day, but that as an averagely gifted musician you need to work much harder, especially if you want to accomplish as much as Heifetz did. This is missing the point. Heifetz was able to make the most of his considerable gifts. The only way in which you can imitate him is by making the most of *your* gifts, whatever they may be. Heifetz was a model of good use, at the violin and away from it. Good use entails reliable sensory awareness, the ability to listen to yourself accurately, and the ability to gauge tension, effort, and movement. Work on your use—with the help of the Alexander Technique—and you will practise more efficiently, thereby better fulfilling your talents. Emulate, then, not the results of Heifetz's practising, but his very way of practising.

Heifetz took frequent breaks in his daily practice. In itself taking breaks is a good idea, but you can turn it into a particularly healthy habit by *working on your use* every time you take a break. Better still, reverse the habit and consider practising during the breaks you may take from working on your use.

Efficient practising entails knowing when to stop. This means when to go from one exercise to the next, when to take a break from practising, and when to stop for the day. If you wish to create a clear kinaesthetic memory of a given gesture, you are better off playing that gesture five times perfectly in a row than nine times perfectly and a tenth time imperfectly, thereby blemishing your memory of the whole set. Similarly, stop the day's work before the onset of fatigue, not after. When practising, create the conditions for you to be at your best. Once you get there, give it up. Remember Alexander: 'The experience you want is in the process of getting it. . . . Getting it, not having it, is what you want.' Quit at your best and your impression of the total practice session will be entirely positive, increasing the likelihood of success the following day. There is truth in the bromide: nothing breeds success like success.

The Objectives of Daily Practice

Before continuing our discussion of the *habits* of daily practice let us define the *objectives* of daily practice. Every musician has his own understanding of why he practises. We saw, for instance, that a musician who repeats the same passage endlessly conceives daily practice as a *search for control*. To improve, to refine, to control, to get it right—these are all avowed objectives of daily practice. None of them, however, addresses the real needs of a musician. William Pleeth writes:

Pablo Casals, by his own account, made a habit of beginning each day by first playing some Bach, to 'sanctify' the house, as he put it. I find this a wonderful idea, for not only does it sanctify the house, but it also sanctifies the mind: the spirit comes in touch with something marvellous, and gives the physical something to ride on. It helps one draw a circle around, or through, the physical and spiritual aspects of one's being and playing so that there is a sense of completeness from the very start.

If you warm up in the right way, all your practising and playing will have a sense of completeness and integration. In the end it is not so much a matter of practising something, but of *living* in a complete way and *then* starting to practise.[24]

We saw in the preceding chapter that (1) the great problem of a musician is to marry technique to content; (2) technique is but applied use of the self; and (3) good use of the self contains within it the seeds of musicality. The objective of daily practice should be to cultivate the best possible use of the self on a general basis, and to apply it correctly on a specific basis, to playing, singing, or conducting.

In other words, working on *right living* should take precedence over working on *right playing*. The objective of daily practice should be for you to make yourself a better person, by working on the use of your whole self. As a consequence you will become a better musician; this in turn will lead you to become a better player. 'As long as we adhere in everything we do to the principle of consciously inhibiting interference with the primary control,' wrote Alexander, 'then our ordinary daily activities can be made a constant means of psycho-physical development in its fullest sense.'[25]

Alexander's words pertain to the subject of warming up. What distinguishes warming up from performing is not the nature of your activity but its degree of complexity. The ideal warm-up is not a series of physical or technical exercises, which would deny the wholeness of your being, but a simpler version of a gesture which affirms your wholeness. Use a scale or arpeggio, for instance, but execute it to principle from the first note onwards: using your whole, co-ordinated self, and infusing the gesture with musicality and rhythmic forward motion.

'The athlete of more advanced years tends to warm up more slowly and for a longer time,' wrote Bruce Lee. 'This fact may be due to greater need for a longer warm-up period, or it may be because an athlete tends to get "smarter" as he gets older.'[26] Norms, which I shall define in Chapter 18, 'Norms and Deviations', make excellent warming-up material. The smarter you become, the more norms you practise.

Alternation, Continuity, and Endurance

Two arguments are sometimes put forth against taking breaks. 'I find stopping disruptive,' goes the first argument. 'If I stop too soon or too often, I lose my train of thought.' 'And if I don't practise a lot and for long periods,' goes the second argument, 'I'll never develop the endurance I need to perform.' Both arguments are fallacious. Alexander told of a writer pupil whose habit of writing for hours at a stretch caused serious health problems. His pupil 'forgot' to take breaks, and claimed too that he lost his train of thought whenever he did stop. Alexander then pointed out that 'it should be as easy to break off a piece of work requiring thought, and take it up again, as it is to carry on a train of thought whilst taking a walk with all its attendant interruptions, and that this should be possible not only without loss of connection, but with accruing benefit to the individual concerned'.[27]

Alexander remarked that the inability to stop during an ordinary activity is symptomatic of the inability to stop generally. It is a lack of control—a failure of inhibition—and therefore an instance of end-gaining. Conversely, Alexander wrote, 'the gaining of control in the simple psycho-physical evolutions in which [an Alexander pupil is] engaged during lessons [means] sooner or later the gaining of control in the practical spheres of his daily life'.[28]

Alternating between different activities in daily practice brings into play mechanisms that might otherwise remain inactive for too long. In ideal use, different sets of muscles all work in a harmonious whole. If a pianist works insistently on a single mechanism—his trills, for instance—he risks both overworking the mechanism in question and underworking other mechanisms, which should all co-operate in the concerted use of the self. His trills will improve faster and more durably if he alternates practising them with other techniques, resting, and working on his use away from the instrument. (Athletes have long accepted that their specialized skills improve when they work on musculatures that are not normally engaged in their particular sport. This is the rationale for cross-training, which is but a manifestation of the principle of alternation.)

'A proper standard of mental and physical perfection', wrote Alexander, 'implies an adaptability which makes it easy for a man to turn from one occupation in which a certain set of muscles are employed, to another involving totally different muscular actions.'[29] It is easy for the well-co-ordinated musician to turn from task to task (or from playing to resting) in his practice. Indeed, this alternating contributes positively to his total co-ordination and well-being.

The second argument against short practising periods concerns endurance. Yet 'fatigue', writes the violinist Carlos Ramos Mejia, 'is a discomfort that cannot be conquered by one's "getting used to it" (as generally accepted amongst violinists), but by eliminating its cause'.[30]

Most often, fatigue is symptomatic not of weakness or lack of endurance, but of misuse of the self. As I wrote in the first chapter, an old African woman can carry heavy weights on her head for long distances, not because of muscular strength but because of her good use. Equally, endurance is but an effect of good use. It should be acquired

indirectly, through good use, rather than directly, though long practising sessions. These have their place in the cycle of alternation, but
as an exception rather than the norm.

Musical Aspects of Alternation

There are purely musical reasons to alternate between activity
and rest, and between different activities. It is outside the scope of this
book to consider all the aspects of alternation in music-making; I mention the following examples to illustrate the universality of the principle.

The study of ear-training, harmony, counterpoint, and music history
is usually undertaken in complete isolation from instrumental techniques and interpretation. Yet surely so-called theoretical knowledge
can and should permeate so-called practical knowledge. By alternating your study of ear-training with scales and arpeggios, for instance,
and scales and arpeggios with running through actual pieces, rather
than studying them all in isolated compartments, you link your ear for
the tonal and harmonic organization of music to your technical abilities. *You begin to hear with your hands*—a marvellous way of improving sight-reading, improvisation, and interpretation.

The mechanisms for playing or singing forte should not be antagonistic, but complementary to those for playing piano. Practising loud
and soft passages in alternation helps you make your technique more
homogeneous. (I shall take up this issue again in Chapter 18, 'Norms
and Deviations'.)

You can practise with a score at the instrument or away from it, or
by heart at the instrument or away from it. Practising in these ways
all in imaginative alternation creates greater freedom than practising
always in one way only. Many other examples will suggest themselves
to you once you appreciate the usefulness of the principle.

On Memory

The memory of a musician is exercised in many different
ways: aural, visual, muscular, verbal, analytical. A detailed study of the

psychology of memory would be outside the scope of this book. I limit my discussion to muscular (or kinaesthetic) memory and to learning and performing music by heart.

Memory has three distinguishable phases: registration, storage, and retrieval. Of the three, registration is the most important, and the one on which the Alexander Technique has greatest direct bearing. The better you register something, the better you memorize it. This is a truism, but it merits our attention.

Alexander wrote of teaching a pupil how to do a whispered 'ah'. 'Before the teacher had finished speaking,' he wrote, 'the pupil was try-ing to memorize [the instructions], as they were given, by a "physical" (sensory) process, i.e. by trying to "feel" the instructions as they were spoken, rather than to acquire them by a process of remembering ("committing to memory," as we say).'[31]

The pupil errs twice. First, he attempts to carry out the instructions before he has understood them. Second, he attempts to register the instructions by feel rather than by listening to them. If his feelings are unreliable, he risks learning something other than what the teacher is trying to teach him. His memory of these instructions will be faint, as he has not really listened to them, and untrustworthy, as what the pupil 'felt' is not necessarily what the teacher said.

To memorize a gesture, first say 'no' to the very wish of memoriz-ing it. Do not act—instead, pay attention to your whole use, and in particular your Primary Control. While *not-acting*, listen, watch, or think, as needed. Then consider the mental commands that the gesture demand, not the feelings that these commands entail. After you have stopped, not-acted, directed your use, listened to the instructions, and memorized the guiding orders, you can try out the gesture and exam-ine how it feels.

You may apply this working principle to all that you wish to memor-ize: a gesture, a technique, a set of instructions, a melody, an operatic role. Let us see how you may commit a score to memory. (Keep in mind that working on your use, a precondition for memorizing scores, does not preclude your using traditional mnemonic tricks, like memor-izing a score from the end to the beginning.)

Do not start playing a new piece from memory too soon, lest you memorize wrong notes. Once you know your score fairly well, use the principle of alternation, and practise with and without music, at the instrument and away from it. The greatest demands are made upon

your memory when you practise away from the instrument and without the score. Place yourself in a position of mechanical advantage,
and, while directing your whole use, hear the score in your mind's ears.
Lie semi-supine, for instance, and leave your score within easy reach.
Run a phrase or section mentally; then, without leaving the position,
take the score in your hands and check your memory for accuracy.
You may also first look at the score, then run a passage mentally.

Some artists have learned and memorized whole scores before ever
playing a note from them. This takes either genius or boundless discipline, but you may attempt it too, starting with short, easy pieces and
building up to more complex ones.

So far I have addressed mostly the subject of registration. About
storage and retrieval, Alexander made an intriguing point:

There can be little doubt that the growing habit of newspaper reading and light
literature, and the accompanying decline in the reading of books or matter which
is to be retained as valuable knowledge, has been accompanied by harmful psycho-
physical habits which today are seriously affecting the human memory, in a degree more or less in accordance with the standard of psycho-physical functioning
of the individual concerned.[32]

We discard much of what we read almost immediately upon having
read it. In the process the abilities to retain, connect, and analyse information suffer, all the more if we misuse ourselves.

Ultimately, memory affects use as much as use affects memory.
Good use is the embodiment of coherence and continuity—between a
thought and an action, from thought to thought, and from action to
action. Alexander wrote:

The employment of inhibition calls for the exercise of memory and awareness,
the former for remembering the procedures involved in the technique and the
proper sequence in which they should be used, and the latter in the recognition
of what is happening. In the process both potentialities are developed, and the
scope of the use of both gradually increased. Moreover, the experiences thus
gained not only help in developing and quickening the recalling and connecting
memory, but cultivate what I shall call the motor-sensory-intellectual memory.[33]

To a certain extent and given the right conditions, the more you have
in your memory, the easier it is to memorize. If you do not have the
habit of playing from memory, the first concerto is daunting. Once
you overcome the inertia of an untrained memory, however, the 'experience makes the meat it feeds on', to use a phrase of Alexander's,
and your memory welcomes new pieces ever more readily and reliably.

Judging Yourself

I started this chapter with a brief consideration of diagnosis. We are ready to reconsider the issue, in light of what we have discussed so far.

You should know what your problems are, how they manifest themselves, what their causes are, what solutions exist, and how to implement them. This all depends on your *knowing yourself* and making an objective, practical assessment of your playing or singing.

Whenever a musician plays for me, I ask him: 'What do you think of how you have just played?' Often a musician's first response is to say, 'I didn't like it.' A little less often someone else says, 'I liked it.' These judgements have little or no value from a practical point of view. What did you like or dislike about your performance, and what do you intend to do about it? These should be your main concerns.

I believe that good assessments go from the general to the particular. Since confidence and freedom go hand in hand, self-assessments should also proceed from the positive to the negative aspects of each performance. To judge your playing and diagnose your problems, then, first establish what aspects of it are healthy and satisfactory, and enumerate these in order of importance. Afterwards, do the same to aspects which seem troublesome and unsatisfactory.

As a convinced Alexandrian, start by considering your use, and above all your Primary Control. What happens to your head, neck, and back when you play or sing? Is your head straight or twisted? Does it contract into the neck, or is it going forward and up, away from the neck? Is your neck free, collapsed, or frozen? Is the joint between the spine and the skull free or locked? Is your spine elastic, slack, or rigid? Is your back lengthening and widening, or shortening and narrowing? Are you twisting your torso? Are you moving or staying still? Are you moving from your joints in the hips, knees, and ankles or by bending at the waist? What happens to your shoulders? Then go on to ask all relevant questions about the arms, hands, fingers, legs, and feet.

You need not ask yourself all questions after every single effort, but you need to have a degree of awareness of what is happening to all these areas of your body at all times. If you prefer you can talk in more general terms, about end-gaining, inhibiting, and directing, concentration and awareness, and the relationship between effort and effect.

After you scrutinize your use from various angles, consider music-making itself. Musical aspects too have their hierarchy. Most musical difficulties are caused by a lack of rhythmic clarity. *Never take rhythm for granted*, and assess your rhythmic precision and forward motion before thinking about intonation, sound-production, or accuracy. Give legato and continuity of musical line priority over right notes, right fingerings, or right words in song. You will soon see that musical continuity is a function of good use, and both together make technical security easier to achieve. Ask yourself if you have shed light on a piece's inner construction before you inspect your ornaments or passage-work.

In sum, proceed from the general to the specific in both diagnosis and remedy. Cultivate practical and objective ways of describing your strengths and weaknesses. Consider your use at all times, with emphasis on the Primary Control. Know your priorities and keep to them. Take time to know what you want to do and how you want to do it. Try to determine if what you conceive, what you do, and what you feel that you do all coincide. And do not think too hard, for goodness' sake.

17 Aesthetic Judgements

Right and Wrong: The What, Why, and How

I help a pupil into a monkey. He objects to it: 'Instinctively I prefer bending my back rather than my knees; it is more natural for me. I couldn't possibly do a monkey in public—people would notice me, and I would lose my spontaneity and become self-conscious.'

In essence the Alexander Technique deals with the way we make judgements of right and wrong, and the relationship between these judgements and our actions. Our mental conceptions of how to do something and the sensations we have while we do it are never separated. 'To act successfully along new lines of thought', wrote Alexander, 'means . . . the carrying-out of a decision . . . not only in the face of our mental conception of HOW that decision should be carried out, but also in the face of real discomfort and "feeling wrong" in carrying it out.'[1]

If only my pupil performed monkeys to principle enough times, he would stop feeling that they are wrong. 'Teaching is like animal training! Make them jump over the stick!' said Giovanni Battista Lamperti. 'Wait for a sign of the pupil's intelligence before giving reasons.'[2] But, precisely because the pupil's sensorial discomfort is inextricably bound up with his intellectual conception of right and wrong, I may have to give him my reasons before I make him jump the stick. My pupil uses many words—'spontaneity', 'natural', 'instinctive'—which I need to discuss before finally proving to him that he is wrong indeed, and that his only choice is to jump the stick.

Normal and Natural

I ask you to sit down or stand up naturally. You understand this to mean 'as you do habitually, without further premeditation'. Similarly, if you are an untrained singer and I ask you to sing me a phrase naturally, you sing to me as you do when you are driving around in your car, or in a crowd in the football ground: in a manner 'marked by easy simplicity and freedom from artificiality, affectation, or constraint' (*Webster's Ninth New Collegiate Dictionary*).

This is a legitimate use of the word 'natural', and yet we should remain aware that it is not the *only* meaning of the word. Alexander pointed out that certain acts and behaviours are considered right or wrong according to circumstance or ever-evolving cultural values; their rightness is therefore relative. Regarding the use of the self, however, Alexander argued that standards of right and wrong are absolute rather than relative. He wrote:

it can be demonstrated that a certain manner of use of the mechanisms is found in association with certain satisfactory standards of functioning and with conditions of health and well-being. We are surely justified in considering a manner of use that is associated with such desirable conditions to be 'natural' or 'right' under all circumstances.[3]

Here Alexander uses 'natural' to mean 'being in accordance with or determined by nature; based on an inherent sense of right and wrong' (*Webster's*). 'Natural', in short, may mean 'unpremeditated' or 'intrinsically right', and unless we specify a meaning when using the word, we risk confusion. This is unwittingly illustrated in a booklet about running: 'Do what comes naturally, as long as "naturally" is mechanically sound. If it isn't, do what is mechanically sound until it comes naturally.'[4]

When my pupil claims that the monkey is not natural, he means that doing a monkey is a strange experience, 'natural' for him being synonymous with 'habitual'. But since what we call 'the monkey' occurs in many situations outside Alexander lessons (in small children at play, among many adults in non-Western cultures and well-co-ordinated adults in Western ones, among martial artists and sportsmen and dancers); since in every instance the monkey is a manifestation of good use and functioning; and since the adult of average co-ordination can learn it easily (thereby improving both his use and functioning), we must consider the monkey truly *natural*—in accordance with the laws of Nature—and therefore intrinsically right.

My pupil claims that it looks funny for him to do the monkey in public. Here he does not offer proof that the monkey is unnatural; rather, he acknowledges a gap between what is intrinsically right and what is socially acceptable.

'One of the most remarkable of man's characteristics', wrote Alexander, 'is his capacity for becoming used to conditions of almost any kind, whether good or bad, both in the self and in the environment, and once he has become used to such conditions they seem to him both right and natural.'[5] Man's adaptability, important as it is for his survival and evolution, also grieves him. In the simple case of the monkey, today it is 'right' to slump, slouch, and twist the back and neck in order to lose height; everybody does it, therefore it is considered 'normal'. Social convention not only allows this misuse; it positively demands it, turning the monkey into a deviation from the norm. 'Contemporaries find it difficult to define the limit of unnaturalness because it coincides with convention,' wrote Wilhelm Furtwängler. 'It is hard to believe how much unnaturalness goes on being swallowed.'[6]

The word 'normal' also has two meanings. If most members of a group act in a certain way—let us imagine that they drink heavily—this behaviour is 'normal' for them ('according to an average'), although not exemplary ('according to an ideal'). Unfortunately, many current standards of taste and behaviour are based on such norms. We all face a constant choice between doing what is right and doing like everybody else.

Nature and Civilization

We use the word 'natural' in a third way. It is frequently said that driving cars (or wearing shoes, sitting in chairs, living in big cities, etc.) is not natural. Yet surely the solution to our problems lies not in moving to the country and growing our own vegetables, but in inhibiting our end-gaining habits, wherever we live, whatever we do. There is a difference between naturalism and naturalness. The first defines 'natural' as everything removed from modern civilization, and is anti-evolutionary and atavistic. The second defines it as 'according to the laws of Nature', and it is evolutionary and forward-looking.

To give an illustration, naturalism sees opera—a contrived art form full of artificial rules—as unnatural, and operatic singing as fabricated and affected. Naturalism calls 'natural' the 'spontaneous' and unaffected singing of the street singer, the mother who sings to her baby, the untrained churchgoer, and so on.

There is no disputing that opera is highly contrived. But the naturalists miss the point entirely. The ideal opera singer is not a freak of nature, someone who sings in an unnatural way. We pay him £20,000 for a night's work because he has fulfilled the nature of his vocal organs—because he is *a marvel of natural functioning in a situation that is admittedly artificial.* The untrained singer sings without affectation, but unnaturally. His voice thus lacks the power, beauty, resilience, flexibility, and virtuosity of the truly natural singer.

As Alexander said, there is an absolute standard of right use of the self, a standard that is adapted and applied to meet *every* circumstance. Opera is in itself unnatural; so are driving cars, reading newspapers, and living in New York City. Yet, there is an intrinsically right way of singing opera and of leading a modern, urban life. You would be closer to Nature by using yourself well in an urban environment than by using yourself badly out in the wild.

Spontaneity, Self-Consciousness, and Self-Awareness

To pass from the known (wrong) to the unknown (right) is an arduous process. A common complaint of the Alexander pupil (and, equally, of the musician who wishes to apply the Technique to music-making) is an apparent loss of spontaneity resulting from his lessons. The pupil finds himself thinking of his actions and gestures all the time. This very examination makes him self-conscious, thereby hindering his gestures. A vicious circle is born.

'I used to be a natural, instinctive musician,' a musician complains. 'I have since lost my spontaneity, and can't play a note without making it laborious and artificial.' He seems to regard naturalness, spontaneity, and instinctiveness as more or less synonymous, and in every case desirable. Let us consider these assumptions. In an Introductory Word to Alexander's *Man's Supreme Inheritance*, the great philosopher and educationalist John Dewey wrote:

The spontaneity of childhood is a delightful and precious thing, but in its original naïve form it is bound to disappear. Emotions become sophisticated unless they become enlightened, and the manifestation of sophisticated emotion is in no sense genuine self-expression. True spontaneity is henceforth not a birthright, but the last term, the consummated conquest of an art—the art of conscious control to the mastery of which Mr. Alexander's book so convincingly invites us.[7]

In a beautiful short story, 'The Marionette Theatre', the German playwright Heinrich von Kleist makes a cogent case for the spontaneity of self-knowledge. The story concludes thus:

We see that in the natural world, as the power of reflection darkens and weakens, grace comes forward, more radiant, more dominating. . . . But that is not all; two lines intersect, separate and pass through infinity and beyond, only to suddenly reappear at the same point of intersection. As we look in a concave mirror, the image vanishes into infinity and appears again close before us. Just in this way, after self-consciousness has, so to speak, passed through infinity, the quality of grace will reappear, and this reborn quality will appear in the greatest purity, a purity that has either no consciousness or consciousness without limit; either the jointed doll or the god. . . . We must eat from the tree of knowledge again and fall back into a state of innocence. . . . That is the last chapter in the history of the world.[8]

In discussing the loss of spontaneity, it may be useful to establish the difference between self-consciousness and self-awareness. While both imply a moment-to-moment measuring of your every action, self-consciousness denotes an uncomfortable, excessive preoccupation with yourself and, above all, with the way others judge you, while in self-awareness this measuring of your actions and of your surroundings is allied to a non-judgemental attitude that allows you to act freely and without undue constraint.

In the journey from the known to the unknown, then, there is a loss of your first spontaneity, the spontaneity of *not knowing*. This is true regardless of how the journey is undertaken, be it through schooling, or the passage of time, or through lessons in the Alexander Technique. Inevitably this loss threatens your well-being and your sense of individuality; all the same, it is a necessary first step on the road to self-awareness.

This applies to all spheres of human endeavour. Some musicians shy away from studying analysis, harmony, counterpoint, history, and so on in the fear that this knowledge might render their performances less spontaneous and moving. This need not be so. The intelligent musician accepts the loss of innocence. If he is particularly talented, he actively pursues it. Claudio Arrau said, 'At a certain moment—at the time of the difficult transition from the intuitive way of playing toward a conscious understanding—I thought of giving up my career. But only for a short time.'[9] I shall return to this point presently.

Instinct and Intuition

Arrau spoke of the 'intuitive way of playing'. Others may call it the instinctive way, or the natural way. We have already considered the word 'natural'. Let us now turn to the difference between instinct and intuition.

In popular usage the two terms are sometimes used interchangeably. Some dictionaries give one as a synonym for the other. Yet they mean distinct things. Alexander wrote: 'I define instinct as the result of the accumulated subconscious psycho-physical experiences of man at all stages of his development, which continue with us until, singly or collectively, we reach the stage of conscious control; whilst intuition is the result of conscious reasoned psycho-physical experiences during the process of our evolution.'[10] H. W. Fowler, the lexicographer, discussed the difference between instinct and intuition briefly in his *Modern English Usage*:

While both, as faculties, are contrasted with that of reason, intuition is the attribute by which gods and angels, saints and geniuses, are superior to the need of reasoning, and instinct is the gift by which animals are compensated for their inability to reason. . . . [Quoting the English essayist and poet Joseph Addison:] 'Our Superiors are guided by Intuition and our Inferiors by Instinct.'[11]

Like Alexander, Fowler put instinct and intuition in evolutionary terms. In our voyage from the known to the unknown—our duty to evolution, so to speak, and 'the last chapter in the history of the world' —we abandon instinct to embrace intuition.

Founded in reason, intuition is subconscious no less—it works reflexively, without the aid of the little man in a lab coat that anti-rationalists imagine reason to be. I liken intuitive subconsciousness to a two-way door. Habits acquired through the Technique—by conscious guidance and control—remain in reach of reason, and can be developed, altered, reshaped, and eliminated at will. *They can be left alone too.* Instinctive subconsciousness, on the other hand, is a one-way door: its habits are permanently out of reach. In intuition, habit is at the service of the individual; in instinct, the individual is slave to habit.

You may analyse Robert Schumann's harmonic language and highlight his chromatically altered chords by acquired habit, reflexively, by *enhanced intuition*, without becoming what some musicians would consider a cold, analytical performer. Similarly, you may study the Alexander Technique and 'think up' by *enhanced intuition*, without seeming less spontaneous than when you pull down.

Note in passing that if we stick to our proposed usage of the words 'instinct' and 'intuition', Arrau really meant 'instinctive' when he spoke of the child-like playing that preceded his mastery of himself.

Originality and Naturalness

Faced with my reasoning, the unreconstructed naturalist may still say, 'Your arguments hold for everyone but me. I like the way I am, and if I go against your immutable laws of Nature, so mch the better: *I am an original* and will enjoy a successful career, as many other originals have done and shall continue to do.'

Let us return to Alexander's statement about absolute standards of right and wrong. In passing from the known to the unknown, I must give up what I perceive as my spontaneity, my instinctive way of playing, my naturalness, ultimately my very sense of self. Indeed, emotionally my use and my identity are one. One of the reasons for my holding on to my way of being is that it helps me believe that I am unlike anybody else. Individuality implies my being separate from the crowd, my being *original*.

By setting down absolute standards of right and wrong use, Alexander affirms that we should all use ourselves in ways that are universal, regardless of sex, race, country of origin, and so on. And yet there is something deeply satisfying about misusing myself. To deviate from a norm makes me stand out from the crowd. In a crooked way, it enhances my sense of self-worth. Above all, it makes me feel as if I am an original.

For Alexander, however, evolutionary duty entails my observing absolute standards of right and wrong use. Yet there need be no conflict between *being like everybody else* and *being myself*. Indeed, the more I follow the dictates of good use (which apply universally), the better I am able to express myself.

Wilhelm Furtwängler addressed this issue too, and established a priority:

Being original means being one's own person, that is, different from the rest. But if everyone is original, as they are today, then no one really is.[12]

There are two mutually contradictory things: originality and naturalness. Anyone who does not have both, who is not and cannot be original and yet natural, natural and yet original and capable, should forget originality. For of the two—and let this be said to our age again and again—naturalness is the more important and the greater thing.[13]

'A good many people, nowadays, confuse gross mal-coordination with originality,' wrote Patrick Macdonald.[14] The Alexander Technique helps you release your true originality, by co-ordinating your whole self along immutable (and utterly unoriginal) laws of Nature. For a well-co-ordinated original, what Furtwängler calls naturalness is the very source of his originality.

Taste, Freedom, and Choice

We started our discussion with the example of a pupil doing a monkey, and proceeded to consider the relationship between a musician's use and his artistic philosophy. Central to the opening argument was my pupil's likes and dislikes. He did not like doing monkeys, and might well argue that there is no disputing taste.

Yet, as Cornelius L. Reid writes, 'most expressions of taste in the form of "like" or "dislike" are bound to be prejudicial almost by definition'.[15] If prejudicial, then they are debatable indeed. Among your likes and dislikes there may be some things that you like despite their being wrong, and, more important, others you may possibly not have the right to like or dislike.

I play the cello in a string quartet. I suggest to the violist that she play a certain long note in one bow. I have valid musical reasons for my request. Before she tries it, and partly as a justification for *not* trying it, she says: 'I don't like that, I prefer playing the note in two separate bow-strokes.' This is a dislike to which she has no right. We all know people who say 'I don't like dancing' who have never danced, or 'I hate oysters' who have never tasted one. Regardless of whether or not my violist agrees with me, *unless she tests something, and until she masters it, she does not have the right to an opinion.*

To be exempt from prejudicial judgements, you have to free yourself from all technical constraints. You cannot claim that you choose to execute a passage the way you do unless you are able to execute it equally well in a whole range of different ways. 'The benefit to be derived from a healthy co-ordinative response', writes Reid, 'is that it provides absolute spontaneity of expression. With the attainment of functional freedom'—what Alexander calls good use of the self—'the singer then becomes able to express *what* he has to say *the way he wants to say it*, not the way he *has* to.'[16]

Functional freedom means being able to execute, freely and convincingly, interpretative choices that you may not particularly like. 'Even though a tone colour produced by a certain type of vibrato might be contrary to the taste of a particular place or time . . . ,' wrote Ivan Galamian, 'the *ability to produce it* cannot become obsolete, and, thus, it has a definite place within the inventory of the absolute values of a complete technical equipment.'[17]

Artistic freedom is inconceivable without functional freedom. To give true expression to your musicality, you must first and foremost have the necessary means at your disposal. 'Functional freedom alone', writes Reid, 'is able to fully release sensitivity, insight, emotional and intellectual depth, and musical perception.'[18] In short, true spontaneity will come to you if you pursue not that which you like, but that which is free.

Interpretation and End-Gaining

Alexander made a distinction between relative standards of right and wrong, such as those that determine cultural and social mores, and absolute ones, such as those that govern the use of the self. This means that a certain behaviour or custom may be considered justifiably right or justifiably wrong by different people, but that a certain use of the self should be considered indisputably right or wrong by all people. Yet, because of the correlation between use and behaviour, we may argue that some behaviours are intrinsically wrong, regardless of time and circumstance, because of the use they engender.

It is logical, then, to ask whether the Alexandrian ideal of use entails an artistic outlook. In other words, is there a way of playing, singing, or conducting that is intrinsically right, by virtue of being associated with an intrinsically right way of using yourself? Would this way of making music be above all considerations of taste? Is public or critical success synonymous with artistic success? What are the differences between an artistic outlook based on the end-gaining principle and

another based on the means-whereby principle? What are the requirements of the latter? How does a musician who is truly free, natural,
spontaneous, intuitive, and self-aware actually sound?

End-gaining manifests itself in all activities. In previous chapters we
saw how it affects musical technique and daily practice. Interpretation,
too, is subject to the consequences of end-gaining. How could it be
otherwise, when technique is inseparable from musicianship?

A saying is attributed to Richard Strauss: it is the audience who
should sweat, not the musician. That is, a musician ought to create
excitement rather than get excited. Musicians end-gain in two ways:
by getting excited, and by creating excitement through means foreign
to the music they perform.

The advice for a musician not to get excited is traditionally given as
'Play with a cold head and a warm heart.' This is wise enough, but an
observation of Cornelius L. Reid's reinvents it in a manner that is perhaps more useful for a convinced Alexandrian: 'Functional freedom
awakens feeling, and when this happens it is not necessary to "put"
feeling into anything. It is there.'[19] In other words, use yourself well
when you make music, and much of your interpretative work is done.
'It is almost self-evident, granted a musical personality,' writes Reid,
'that all tones truly free are either beautiful or legitimately expressive.'[20]

To 'put feeling' into your performances is to end-gain. Feeling
should arise of its own, through the freedom of the technique and the
substance of the music itself. To succeed in letting feeling exist, rather
than willing it into existence, you need to observe a few guidelines.

In the previous chapter I spoke of rhythmic discipline and forward
motion in music-making. These two qualities are indispensable both
to free your technique and to make it pregnant with musical meaning.
As for beauty of tone, use yourself as well as you can, and your tone
will be as free as it can be. If you seek freedom, beauty will arrive of
its own. But if you seek beauty directly, you risk losing freedom *and*
its attendant beauty.

Contemplate now the relationship between a musician and music
itself. I said earlier that it is end-gaining to produce excitement by
means foreign to the music itself. This happens when a musician's personality obscures or overpowers the work of art.

'Every work carries within it its own "distance", from which one
must consider it', wrote Furtwängler. 'To discover this distance and
act accordingly is the principal duty of the performer.'[21] It is this distance that allows great musicians to reveal to the public the unfolding

of a piece's structure. Nadia Boulanger recounts an instructive anecdote:

One day [the French pianist Alfred] Cortot confided to me:

'Do you know, you once said something that has touched me more than anything else? It was twenty years ago, I had just played Chopin's *Preludes* and you came . . .'

'Ah! I remember,' I interrupted him.

After a concert in which he had played the *Preludes*, I'd been to see him in his dressing-room and declared, 'A lot of people are asking me for my opinion, to described how you played. I have no idea. All I know is that I've never found the *Preludes* so beautiful.'

He had focused all his light on the *Preludes*, not the other way around. I had heard the work in all its splendour. My forgetting the interpreter wasn't neglect, on the contrary. It put him very high, because the light of someone who is nothing illuminates nothing.[22]

'It is not, "I am doing this," ' wrote Bruce Lee, 'but rather, an inner realization that "this is happening through me", or "it is doing this for me." '[23] To put feeling into your music-making, to get excited, to emote, to use outlandish tempos and dynamics and articulations, to use exaggerated slides and capricious rubatos, to linger upon details at the expense of the whole may gratify the musician. But he would be missing something infinitely more satisfying. Nadia Boulanger said:

I have always preferred the word 'transmit' to 'interpret', it seems to take better account of the attitude necessary to those whose job is to shed light on a work. . . . In my opinion, once the interpreter takes over, the game becomes unbalanced. The interpreter gains, but the work loses. A sublime interpretation is essentially one which makes me forget the composer, forget the interpreter, forget myself; I forget everything except the masterpiece.[24]

Stage Choreography

We call the sum total of a man's gestures, tics, and facial expressions his 'body language'. For the purposes of this discussion I shall call it 'choreography'. A performer's choreography is an integral part of his music-making. It has many characteristics, not all of which are manifestations of the same thing. It can be spontaneous or cultivated, conscious or unconscious, detrimental or beneficial.

Necessary movement is healthy by definition. Unnecessary movement, however, is harmless at best and harmful at worst. Frowning, for instance, is a common mannerism, but in most cases it does no harm to a musician's technical freedom. A musician who uses himself well—whose spine is neither slack nor contracted, and whose head, neck, and back work harmoniously—may shake his head and nod, vigorously even, without interfering with his technique. His head movements may not be needed, but they are not necessarily harmful. A musician who misuses himself, however, contracts his head into his spine whenever he shakes his head or nods, with reverberations throughout the whole organism. His head movements are both unneeded and harmful.

Much of choreography is simply symptomatic of a faulty technique. 'All essential movement [in singing]', writes Reid, 'is interior movement and, as such, should not involve exterior muscular tension. Visible external muscular activity indicates interference, and compensatory gestures only add to that interference rather than serving to alleviate it. Physical evidence of work is tantamount to struggle.'[25]

This is self-evident for singers, but it applies equally to other musicians. 'A pianist who is unable to render musical expression without hysterics or cramps', wrote Neuhaus, 'will inevitably have a hysterical and cramped, in other words an imperfect, technical mechanism and the main components of music—time (rhythm) and tone—will be perverted and distorted.'[26]

Choreography caused by faulty technique cannot be justified. Indeed, it *becomes* faulty technique, and exaggerates the misuse for which it originally compensates. Further, most musicians who misuse themselves are unaware of their harmful mannerisms, and cannot therefore speak of their style as a conscious choice.

Interestingly, a musician often feels that his extraneous gestures are not only technically necessary but also an integral part of his interpretations. Unless he moves so, he believes that his singing will be inexpressive or boring. Here again we see the inseparability of technique and musicianship, as well as the emotional identification we all have with the way we use ourselves. Overcoming technical deficiencies may entail the loss of some precarious inner balance: things will get worse before they get better.

Most of the finest artists in music history have always performed with total detachment and self-effacement, and driven their audiences to rapturous heights on the strength of their musical insights alone. It is surprising, then, that there are musicians of solid musical authority who, rather than relying on their abundant artistry, are compelled to infuse their performances with all manners of superfluous gestures, grimaces, and grunts, either because they lack belief in their own authority or because they underestimate their audiences. Their unnecessary mannerisms may not impair their music-making, but they diminish their artistic dignity—public success notwithstanding. The public is capable of appreciating the self-effacement of a great musician; witness the triumphs of Artur Rubinstein, Claudio Arrau, Carlos Kleiber, and others. Yet it is equally capable of responding enthusiastically to an end-gaining, exhibitionistic performer. In the first case, public success coincides with artistic success. In the second, public success means that an exhibitionistic performer has found his voyeuristic audience.

Le stricte nécessaire should be your motto, in technique and musicianship. Yet you have a duty even to those audiences who positively demand exaggerated choreography from a performer. To satisfy such an audience's thirst, do a little more than necessary, but choose to do more of what is good, right, and free. 'From the technical point of view', wrote the pianist Gyorgy Sandor, 'slow and flexible extra motions may be of value, whether they are instinctive or consciously cultivated.'[27] A pianist who shakes her head vigorously or hollows her back may arouse an audience but harm herself. If, however, she moves from side to side, or leans forwards and backwards from the hip-joints while keeping the relationship between the head, neck, and back constant, she may captivate the visually oriented members of the public without damaging her use or her music-making. Indeed, to move thus is an excellent way of fighting what Sandor called 'negative mannerism', the stage rigidity caused by fear or timidity.

Let us conclude this chapter by celebrating human diversity, whether manifested in 'body language', taste, personality, or musicianship. Alfred Cortot's is not the only way to interpret Chopin. Simply, it is closer to the Alexandrian ideal of *non-doing* than interpretations which cater to the public's intemperate tastes. We should all be grateful for the wealth of artistic conceptions that the world has always known. As committed Alexandrians, we should be more grateful still for the means that exist for us to discern, understand, and actualize the most precious of these conceptions.

18 Norms and Deviations

Norms and Deviations Defined

In a lesson, the Alexander teacher aims to give you ideals of movement, gesture, thought, and direction. Let us call them norms of good use: 'authoritative standards, models' (*Webster's Ninth New Collegiate Dictionary*). A norm is the way you should use yourself optimally. Your habitual misuse is a deviation from the norm.

It is easier to embody these ideals in the hands of an Alexander teacher, in the protected environment of the teaching-room, than in the outside world, under the stress of daily life. Similarly, as a musician you may stick to norms of good music-making in the practice room but deviate from them under the stress of performance. The clearer you make your norms, the easier you will find it not to deviate from them.

Thinking in terms of norms and deviations helps us understand the logic of Alexander's work. It is also an eminently practical way of solving problems. Alexander's whole technique came about as he tried to solve a specific problem—the hoarseness from which he suffered as a young Shakespearean recitalist. After he set out to discover the causes of his hoarseness, he realized that his reciting deviated from his ordinary manner of speaking. Later on, he came to the conclusion that his speech itself deviated from ideals of use. Before working on his reciting, he needed to work on his speech; before working on his speech, he needed to work on his whole use. Alexander took the argument further, and established a general principle:

The attainment of any desired end ... involves the direction and performance of a *connected series of preliminary acts* by means of the mechanisms of the organism. ... These preliminary acts, though means, are also ends, but not isolated ends, inasmuch as they form a co-ordinated series of acts to be carried out 'all together, one after the other.'[1]

To accomplish an act, you must beforehand effectively learn all its component acts. Mastery depends on your not deviating from any of the norms which, together and in succession, make up any given gesture.

The principle of norm and deviation is pertinent to all human endeavour. You may apply it to the cultivation of good use in general, and also to your music-making. In your daily practice, establish norms of sound, rhythm, intonation, articulation, and accuracy; on the concert-platform, prevent all deviations from these norms.

Norms of good use and of music-making are closely related; to work on one is to work on the other. The lunge, for instance, is a norm of postural behaviour from which the flautist or violinist ought not to deviate as she performs a concerto. The hands-on-the-back-of-the-chair establishes norms for the use of the arms, wrists, hands, and fingers which the cellist or pianist ought to apply to her playing at all times. A singer uses the whispered 'ah' to establish norms of freedom and co-ordination for her neck, lips, tongue, and jaw; these norms established, she then inhibits all deviations from them, in speech and in song.

Norms specific to music-making (rhythm, articulation, etc.) are never divorced from norms of use of the self. The latter precede and contain the former: the better you use yourself, the better you will sing or play. Let us discuss norms and deviations first in connection to applied use, then in connection to specific aspects of music-making.

Cultivate Norms, Inhibit Deviations

Consider a flautist of average co-ordination. When playing the flute she twists her torso and shortens it on the right side; lifts her shoulders and brings the right shoulder forwards and the left backwards; twists her head on the neck, to the right and down; hollows her back; lifts her shoulders with each breath; takes her head back and down with each breath and each attack; gasps audibly with each breath; emphasizes accents by shortening the back; and keeps time by nodding, by tapping her feet, or by bending and unbending her legs.

Each of these misuses is a deviation from norms of good use. In ideal conditions, lifting your arms need not and should not cause you to raise, twist, and contract your shoulders. Bringing the flute to your mouth need not and should not cause you to twist your head and contract your neck. Taking breaths need not and should not cause you to gasp, lift your shoulders, or throw your head back and down. Let us see, then, what you could do about these misuses.

1. Start by putting the flute away. Before you do anything with your arms, direct your head, neck, back, and legs, thereby cultivating *norms of good use without the use of the arms.*

2. Now lift your arms in front you, each in turn and both together, at different speeds and heights, angles, and distances one from the other, in pronation and in supination, with wrists in or wrists out, with hands open or closed, in alternation and in combination. Observe yourself in front of the mirror; use your hands and arms against a wall; put your hands on the back of a chair; do all of the above in a monkey or in a lunge. Start with easy gestures and increase the complexity and difficulty of combined gestures. Cultivte *norms for the use of the arms without the flute*, being sure throughout to inhibit all deviations from the norms you established earlier, when you worked on the use of head, neck, back, and legs alone.

3. Now take the flute in your hands. Bring it up to your mouth without attempting to play; do so in different speeds and to different angles, and cultivate *norms for holding the flute without playing it,* inhibiting with every gesture all deviations to previously established norms.

4. Now start cultivating *norms for playing the flute,* by playing single notes, then scales and simple passages, then complete phrases and passages. Each step creates its own norms, and ought not to deviate from any previous step. If ever you deviate, backtrack and re-cultivate earlier norms until a new step does not compromise earlier ones.

This method proceeds from the general to the particular, and is applicable to all musicians in all situations. It is outside the scope of this book to catalogue every difficulty and its many solutions, but I should like to give a few examples of typical misuses, and invite you to imagine ways of cultivating right norms in each case.

- The cellist twists his torso from left to right; lifts and advances shoulders; shortens his spine for all changes of left-hand position; sits slumped against the back of the chair, lower back hollowed, heels off the ground; squeezes the cello with his legs; twists his head around to look at his left hand, or to avoid pushing his head into the pegs; keeps time by nodding.
- The pianist slumps at the piano and brings her head down when

looking at the keyboard; lifts her shoulders and throws her head downwards first, then backwards with every attack; twists her torso to move her hands across the keyboard.

- The singer lifts her shoulders and gasps with every breath; curves her back, contracts her entire torso, and tightens her arms and hands; tightens her legs and feet; sways her body sideways, forwards, and backwards to keep time.

Before you read on, study the photographs of the violist William Primrose (Fig. 22a–c). As he sat, as he stood, as he played at the tip of the bow, as he used left hand and left shoulder to support the instrument (all of which you can see in the photos), never did he deviate from norms of good use. You may wish to hear the results of his discipline on a CD, entitled 'William Primrose'.[2]

Building-Blocks

Heinrich Neuhaus writes of solving difficulties at the piano: 'As a rule difficulties are overcome by splitting up the work to be done, in other words by making the problem easier. . . . With a certain amount of thought everything "difficult," complicated, unfamiliar, inaccessible, can be reduced to something much more easy, simple, familiar, attainable.'[3]

The violinist Carlos Ramos Mejia gives the example of the staccato, which consists of light, short, fast, separated bow-strokes, presenting problems of co-ordination for many pupils. For Mejia, to master the staccato you need first to conquer the separate motions which together make it up:

In bow strokes . . . there exist movements of a simple nature, and of a composite nature. The staccato is undoubtedly an important difficulty as it is composed of a number of movements of unlike nature. The mastery of this bow stroke depends, therefore, on that of each separate movement, the ensemble of movements unified eventually in a single complex movement and triggered by a single act of the will. What would be the point, then, of working continuously on special staccato exercises if the détaché hasn't been dominated, or if the legato is imperfect, or if the bow lacks the necessary stability on the string?

The difficulty of the staccato can be overcome by the great majority of players. Yet one can be assured that its mastery is dependent upon the partial mastery of all the bow-strokes that constitute the mechanism of the right arm.[4]

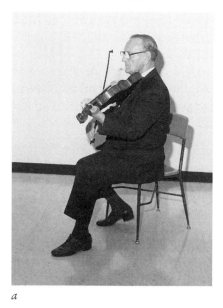

a

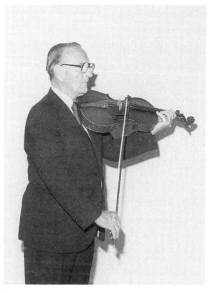

b

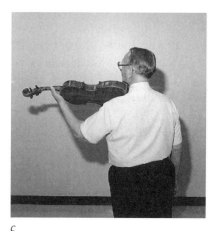

c

FIG. 22. William Primrose at the viola

Neuhaus, too, considers piano playing from this perspective, and enumerates the building-blocks of technique in increasing order of complexity: the single note, groups of two to five notes, scales, arpeggios, double notes, the chord, leaps, and polyphony.

Phrases and passages usually contain several elements combined.

Using our present framework, we may say that technical and musical mastery entails establishing norms of freedom and beauty for the simplest building-blocks, and preventing all deviations from these norms as you put the blocks together in a harmonious whole. In daily practice, perfect the building-blocks on their own first, in combinations of increasing complexity later, and as they occur in actual music-making later still.

Norms and Learning Repertoire

Practising scales and arpeggios is akin to acquiring a vocabulary in order to construct sentences and paragraphs. Although many musicians practise scales and arpeggios as a matter of course, they tend to play them in a perfunctory manner, believing perhaps that they are but finger exercises without musical content or worth. They also tend to isolate their scales and arpeggios from the studying of their repertoire, as if one had no bearing upon the other.

In Chapter 15, 'Technique', I pleaded that you infuse your whole practice with the utmost musicality; in Chapter 17, 'Aesthetic Judgements', I argued that it is not necessary to fabricate musicality or overlay it upon technique. Let us see how to bring both ideas together, with the help of norms and deviations. Consider Ex. 18.1.

Learning a melody is like building a pyramid. At the base there are the various scales and arpeggios, whole or fragmented, which combine to form the melody; at the top, there is the melody itself. Your pyramid needs solid foundations. If your scales and arpeggios are effortless and luminous, so will be your arias and songs.

1. Before you sing anything, take time to think about your use. Heighten your awareness of head, neck, and back. Look for the support in the legs and back that allows the neck and shoulders to be free. Do not restrict your breathing, or force it. Get rid of all hesitation and eagerness, and assume an attitude of non-judgemental, *disinterested interest*.

2. Start by singing a single note, on one of the vowels basic to all singing: 'ah' or 'ee'. (Ex. 18.2). If when singing this note you lose some of the norms of good use you cultivated earlier, go back to the first step and nourish yet again the upward and outward directions which

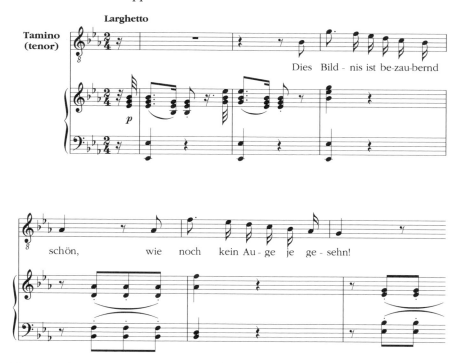

Ex. 18.1. From W. A. Mozart, *Die Zauberflöte*, Act I: Tamino's aria 'Dies Bildnis ist bezaubernd schön'

Ex. 18.2

should precede and accompany everything you do. Eventually you will become comfortable with all vowels on all pitches, but first establish norms of beauty and freedom on these easier vowels, and then inhibit all deviations from such norms on other vowels.

3. Once you can sing a single note with complete freedom, you may proceed to an arpeggio, in which all notes should sound as free as the single note you worked on earlier (Ex. 18.3). Work on a variety of vowels, always starting with those that help you set authoritative standards for all vowels.

4. Sing an arpeggio again, but now take it higher (Ex. 18.4). If there is a deviation—a note out of tune, a loss of brilliance or ease, a wobble

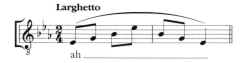

Ex. 18.3

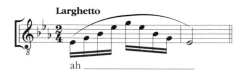

Ex. 18.4

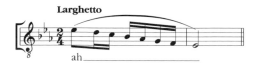

Ex. 18.5

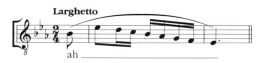

Ex. 18.6

or a jerk, a stiffening of the neck and shoulders, a change of heart—go back a step or two, and wait to resume your advance until you have cleared your mind's ears from all flawed sounds, be they heard, anticipated, or feared.

5. Go on to a new norm: a descending scale (Ex. 18.5). Keep in mind throughout that you are not 'pushing the right buttons' or 'pressing the right leverages'; rather, you are making music. Your every note, scale, and arpeggio ought to compel an observer to sit up and listen to you attentively.

6. Begin to combine different norms—for the use of your whole self, for a single note, for a scale, for an arpeggio—in a form that resembles Mozart's melody, without being as demanding, musically and technically, as the melody itself (Ex. 18.6). Resist the ever-greater temptations to end-gain and deviate.

7. Take your scale closer to Mozart's melody, still singing on an easy vowel (Ex. 18.7).

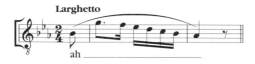

Ex. 18.7

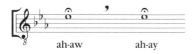

Ex. 18.8

$\frac{2}{4}$ Dies Bild - nis ist be-zau-bernd schön,   wie noch kein Au-ge je ge-sehn!

Ex. 18.9

8. Before going on, take a different tack for a while: sing a sustained single note again, but over changing vowels. Attempt easier changes first—from 'ah' to 'aw', for instance, or from 'ah' to 'ay' (Ex. 18.8). Once you can do that without interfering with the continuity of the vocal line, try the sequence of vowels that Mozart's text requires.

9. Before you sing the melody wholly as Mozart wrote it, establish norms of speech clear enough not to be disturbed by singing. Direct your neck, head, back, lips, tongue, and jaw. Execute a few whispered 'ah's. Then speak Mozart's text, unmeasured first and then in the rhythm of the melody (Ex. 18.9).

10. You have reached the summit of the pyramid. You are now ready to sing Mozart's aria with the mastery it both requires and deserves. If you fail to do it justice on a first attempt, go back to some of the preceding norms and try again. If you sing it perfectly once, go back a few steps all the same before singing it a second or third time.

You may argue that this method is reductionist and mechanical, and that to go through it is a long, boring, and unnecessary process. Why not approach Mozart's music directly and sing it simply and with feeling?

The method I propose develops both 'technique' and 'interpretation', and when the procedure is well carried out there is no separation between the two. There is an organic logic to the way the steps follow one from the other. It has been said that what matters is not how fast you go but how soon you get there. Even if there are ten or more steps to this procedure, it is a much shorter way to mastery and freedom—the desired end—than simply repeating the whole phrase again and again, without an awareness of how it is constructed, or of how you use yourself as you sing it. In any case, by successfully performing all steps leading to a particular phrase you cultivate many norms which recur in subsequent phrases, which you can then practise in lesser detail. As Alexander said, 'a person who learns to work to a principle in doing one exercise will have learned to do all exercises'.[5]

Boring it may seem, but not to an artist or a thorough professional. 'To become a champion,' wrote Bruce Lee, 'requires a *condition of readiness* that causes the individual to approach with pleasure even the most tedious practice.'[6] The better you use yourself, the more you will enjoy the discipline of simplicity.

Last but not least, every one of the steps you take along this path heightens your awareness of the way you use yourself. Norms of use and norms of music-making become intertwined, and working on yourself and working on music-making become one and the same. We may restate Keats's saying that 'beauty is truth, truth beauty' as 'beauty is freedom, freedom beauty'. Use the concept of norms and deviations to free your singing, and Mozart's beauty will shine of its own.

Structure and Ornament

You need not limit the concept of norms and deviations to working on the scales and arpeggios hidden in musical passages. In the phrase from the cello literature quoted in Ex. 18.10, the technical difficulty lies in playing the quavers and the appoggiatura cleanly and easily. First conceive of the passage's barest outline, then add details and embellishments one by one, *in order*, until you reach the passage as Beethoven wrote it (Ex. 18.11). Spend more time on the simpler versions of the passage, and master each version before going to the next. Practise with ever-present rhythmic precision and drive. Notice where the difficulties lie as you progress from simplicity towards complex-

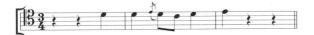

Ex. 18.10. From L. van Beethoven, Sonata for piano and cello in A major, Op. 69, Scherzo: Allegro molto

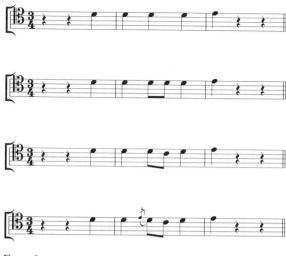

Ex. 18.11

ity, and direct your use accordingly. If you follow these guidelines, you will master this particular difficulty in the shortest possible time, gain confidence, and make further obstacles ever easier to overcome. Remember that all of music derives from the simplest elements; you can apply the above procedure to your entire repertoire, *as needed.*

For this practice to be effective, however, it is not enough to cultivate norms to the letter. Frank Merrick writes:

Some publications . . . preface the pieces with preliminary exercises or special advice as to how to overcome the difficulties. The exercises are all too often mere variants of the figures presenting technical difficulty and rarely develop the student's perception of the musical meanings of the piece. It would be better if the latter consideration were always kept to the fore.[7]

Good use, musical desire, and great rhythmic precision and forward motion should suffuse your every gesture. The component parts must be likenesses of the whole, otherwise you will not be cultivating true norms of freedom.

Loud and Soft, Fast and Slow, and Other Norms

As I noted earlier, the principle of norms and deviations applies to all aspects of music-making. This includes sound, dynamics, and tempo. Remember the *Webster's* definition: norms are 'authoritative standards, models'. There is a model of sound, to be cultivated in preference to and in precedence over other sounds. The following writer, for instance, believes that this norm is *soft*: 'It's much better to sing new material softly, allowing the desired volume to blossom naturally. In order for you to create this same sensation, you must sing as softly as possible yet still resonantly.'[8] This is a commonly held view, which I believe mistaken. The true norm for sound is *loud*, writes Cornelius L. Reid: 'As a general rule, correct soft singing represents the art of producing the voice, and its consistent use is inadvisable until the final stages of technical development. To develop a student's vocal potential, emphasis should be placed on building, not restraining.'[9]

Soft singing is not a legitimate way of acquiring a vocal technique; rather, it is an ability dependent upon acquired vocal technique. To put it differently, you can do greater harm to your voice by singing badly and softly than by singing badly and loudly. Simply, you are more likely to achieve vocal freedom if you sing loudly at first.

In Chapter 10, 'The Arms and Hands', we saw how, at the cello or the piano, forte dynamics require less muscular tension than piano. This is a universal principle. Leon Goossens and Edwin Roxburgh write about oboe playing: 'Throughout the early stages of playing the pupil should always be encouraged to play with a full tone. In developing control of muscles for embouchure and breath-support a sense of vigour will encourage the maturing of control and projection. . . . A strong, firm sound must be the basis for all extremes of dynamics.'[10]

Similarly in flute playing: according to Nancy Toff, the French flautist Marcel Moyse suggests that 'the jaw should be slightly tense for soft passages and quite slack in loud ones, just as the lips should be slightly tighter for softer passages, less for fortes'.[11] Singing, then, is no exception to this rule.

The principle of norms and deviations applies to matters of motion and speed too. Compare the scales in Ex. 18.12. Dynamic balance is more easily achieved than static balance. For most musicians, and particularly for beginners, the first scale is harder to play freely than the second one, just as it is harder to learn how to ride a bicycle slowly. The norm of daily practice should be *moderately fast work*, not slow as most people believe.

Here I recall the principle of alternation, discussed in Chapter 16, 'Daily Practice'. In intelligent practice, you alternate playing loudly and softly, fast and slow, big sweeping gestures and small ones—always

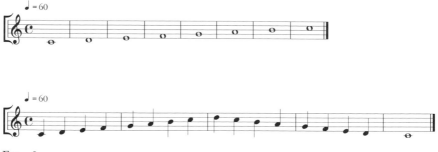

Ex. 18.12

putting an emphasis on loud, moderately fast, and sweeping. 'Since confidence is the prerequisite of freedom,' wrote Heinrich Neuhaus, 'it is confidence that one should stubbornly strive for.'[12] 'Playing should be intense, strong, loud, deep and precise.'[13]

The rule of daily practice is to simplify passages, work on norms, and inhibit deviations. The opposite method, however, has its merits too. Make a problem harder, by increasing its musical and technical complexities or by further challenging your co-ordination as you perform the passage in question. If you can juggle and ride a unicycle at the same time, then juggling or riding alone should be pretty easy.

Neuhaus the dialectician pionts out that this is an antithesis to the thesis of cultivating norms. It makes practising complete. To be truly effective, however, it should play a secondary role in your daily work, and always in alternation with the standard method of breaking down difficulties.

Finally, you can use the practice of norms both to improve your last-minute concert preparation and to lessen stage fright. It is a truism of musical pedagogy that it is too late to learn a piece on the eve of a performance. If you find yourself playing frantically through hard passages backstage before a concert, you have not done your homework properly. Regardless of your state of preparedness, the best thing to do immediately before a concert, and in the days leading up to it, is to practice not hard passages, but the norms underlying these passages. To play a hard passage is to work on a problem; to practice norms is to work on a solution. Practising norms is timeless: even in the greenroom and during the interval, it remains healthy to work on them.

Stage fright is a multi-headed beast, and we shall study it in Chapter 23, 'Stage Fright'. Here let us agree that working on norms lessens the likelihood of stage fright, while deviating from them increases it.

19 *Delayed Continuity*

Thinking up in Silence

In your Alexander beginnings, you may find it difficult to think up and play at the same time. You start playing determined to think up, only to find that there seems not to be enough *time* in between all the notes for you to carry on thinking up.

There are two different but connected challenges in the Alexander Technique. The first is to learn how to think up along the spine; the second is to do it all the time, in every situation. Indeed, if you cannot think up when you sing or play, your thinking up is nearly useless. The greater Alexander challenge, then, is to think up in action, not separately from it.

When you learn a foreign language, you may again find it difficult at first to say whole phrases correctly; after a word or two you get lost for words, you make grammatical mistakes, your diction fails you, your accent becomes more pronounced. If, however, you construct the whole phrase in your mind before you open your mouth, and if you have enough time in between words to remind yourself of what you want to say and how you want to say it, then you will certainly speak clearly and correctly.

Syntax, diction, intention, and good use of the self all carry a phrase forwards in the absence of actual vocal continuity. When Dr Martin Luther King Jr. spoke, for instance, he held the attention of his listeners even when he paused between words or sentences.

In music too you can play deliberately, and pause between notes or melodic fragments. Use yourself well, play each segment with rhythmic precision and forward motion, let your silences be impregnated with musical intention, and you will hold the attention of your listeners whether you play or remain silent.

If you use your silences to inhibit and direct, eventually your upward thought becomes ever-present and continuous. You will then think up in rest and in motion, in sound and in silence. This is the

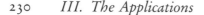

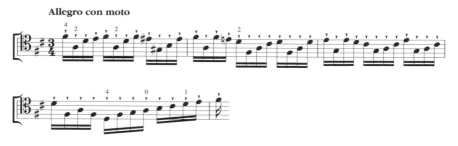

Ex. 19.1. From Adrien-François Servais, Caprice Op. 11 No. 2

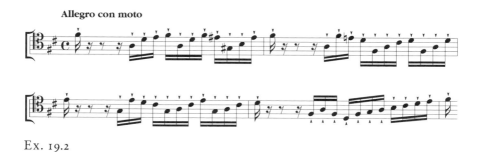

Ex. 19.2

purpose of *delayed continuity*—the practice of inserting silences in phrases, without losing the continuity of musical thought and forward motion.

Silent Anticipation

Let us consider Ex. 19.1. The staccato bow-stroke (fast, short notes with a bouncing bow) is difficult to play evenly and cleanly, and in co-ordination with the left hand. In this passage the difficulty is compounded by the change of string every few notes: there has to be an adjustment in right-arm height for every string crossing, which may disrupt the evenness of the bow-stroke.

Write in a one-beat rest after the first note in each bar. Then use this silence to direct your whole self and adjust your arm for the first string crossing (Ex. 19.2). Your short-term muscular memory of the first, successful string crossing will take care of the next few crossings. By stopping once every few crossings, you keep your muscular memory of success ever fresh. Soon you find that you do not need to stop every bar: a single successful crossing allows you to carry on for several bars. Later, you can do several lines in succession, and finally the whole étude.

This exercise, like all others, is only useful if you perform it to principle. At first you may find that the rests you create in each measure hinder your playing, rather than help it. This happens when you do not use the silence to inhibit and direct. Think of the difference between a puppy dog that has irrepressible urges to move, run, yelp, or simply wag his tail, and a prize-winning guard dog that stands still as long as his master so demands of him, regardless of whatever stimulation comes his way. For your silences to be effective, you need to be able to resist the temptations of end-gaining.

You need to separate the directions that you give yourself to prepare an action from the consent you give yourself to act. In other words, be able to command your elbow to prepare a string crossing without letting the elbow move or contract in any way. Intently fighting your eagerness to go on is futile; rather, you must simply *not wish to go on* until the time is right. Use your silences constructively, with calm, intelligence, and clarity of purpose. Do not freeze into stiff immobility; be ready to move but willing to wait. Do not hurry, do not misuse your head, neck, and back, do not hold your breath, and do not wag your tail.

You may alter the metre of the passage by adding one or more beats of silence per bar, but you must adhere strictly to its pulse. Good use is characterized by good rhythm and enhanced by it; the more rhythmic your playing, the freer it becomes. Good rhythm entails forward motion, a phenomenon exceedingly difficult to describe. In Ex. 19.2, you can make the passage technically more secure and musically more compelling by creating or projecting a forward motion from the beginning of each segment to the first note of the bar that follows it.

During the silence, renew your primary directions and send your secondary and tertiary directions. In other words, pay attention first and foremost to head, neck, and back; then to shoulders and arms; then to wrists and fingers. This may seem quite a lot to think of in a pause that lasts less than a second. Yet, just as a flash of end-gaining thought is enough to disco-ordinate the whole self, a flash of upward thought may be enough to co-ordinate the whole self. Further, if all is as it should be, the primary directions are only inhibitory. You need not *do* anything to head, neck, and back; rather, *stop or prevent doing* all that is excessive or needless. In time you will *stay* up effortlessly before, during, and after the silences. You can then use the pauses simply to observe, feel, and enjoy the continuity of musical line that exists in suspended action.

An instrumentalist who practises delayed continuity has two choices during her silences. The first is to pause in the position in which she finds herself at the end of a segment; the second is to move quickly into the position that starts the following segment, and pause in this new position until the end of the silence. Good use and technical freedom demand that you be comfortable with both methods, and that you pass easily from one to the other.

Silent Rehearsal

You may create silences long enough to fit in a phrase, in whole or in part, and then use the silences to think through the segment in your mind's ears before performing it. Consider the melody shown in Ex. 19.3.

Singing makes numerous demands on the singer. Intonation, clarity of diction, vocal production, rhythmic stability, dramatic content, as well as the use of the whole self, all have to be considered. Lose control of one or more of these aspects, and soon you start compensating for the loss in some way. Compensation creates its own problems, and before long you get ever smaller results for ever greater efforts.

Delayed continuity helps you build up the ability to attend to all aspects at the same time, over the whole phrase, by breaking up a phrase into shorter segments, more easily managed. Musical logic should dictate the choice of breaking-points. Some choices present themselves readily; the phrase in Ex. 19.4 has many places where a break may be created. Other phrases may demand thoughtful experimentation.

As for the length of silences inserted before each segment, you have two choices. First, make the silence as long as the segment, and use it to run the segment once in your mind's ears. Second, increase the number of silent rehearsals. If a segment has four beats, add two or more groups of four beats. Think twice, sing once. Think thrice, sing once. Think ten times, sing once. You will be surprised at how difficult it is to inhibit your desire to skip the silent rehearsal and go on with the performance.

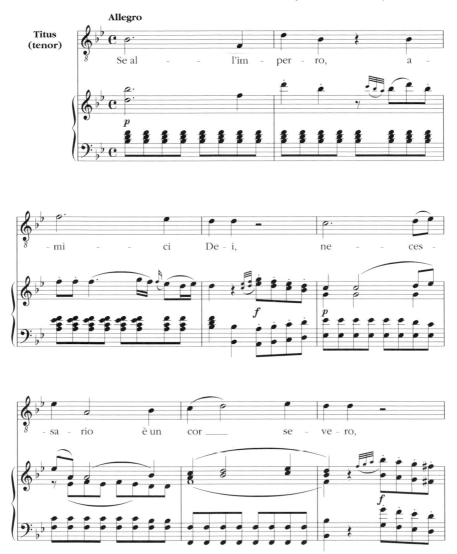

Ex. 19.3. From W. A. Mozart, *La clemenza di Tito*, Act II, Scene i: Tito's aria 'Se all'impero, amici Dei!'

Allegro

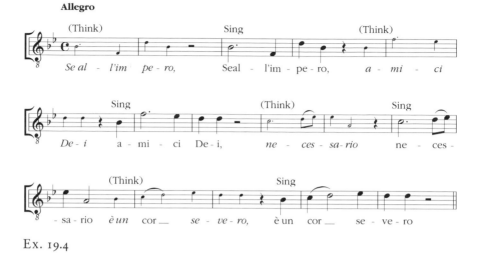

Ex. 19.4

Every time you practise delayed continuity, you have the choice of adding a single beat, two or more beats, or one or more silent rehearsals. Alternate freely between various lengths of silence and no silence at all. You may change the metre and tempo of a passage, but keep its pulse steady. At times the composer writes in a change of tempo, an accelerando or ritardando, a fermata. Whenever you change the pulse or the tempo of a passage, make sure that you do so out of musical choice or need, rather than out of technical inadequacy. To prove to yourself that your changes are not determined by faulty technique, play a passage to perfection and metronomically before you alter its tempo or speed in any way.

20 *Variables and Constants*

A Definition

If all things changed all the time, there would be chaos. If nothing ever changed, there would be no life. And so in music. In every composition, from Gregorian chant to Italian opera, from Mozart to Boulez, the interplay of elements that change and elements that stay the same provides the very essence of the piece. Take opening of the Prelude in C major from the first volume of Johann Sebastian Bach's *Well-Tempered Clavier* (Ex. 20.1).

The pulse, metre, and rhythm are all constant. The contour of the arpeggio is constant: always ascending, with pitches placed at intervals that vary relatively little. The articulation remains constant. These are all building-blocks that change little for the entire duration of the prelude. A single element differentiates one bar from the next: a change of harmony and a corresponding change in pitch and fingering.

Let us call each building-block a *variable*. Pulse, metre, rhythm, contour, articulation, harmony are all variables. In Ex. 20.1, there is a single change of a single variable per bar. All other variables remain constant throughout the bar and beyond it.

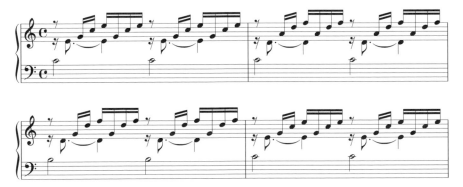

Ex. 20.1. From J. S. Bach, Prelude in C BWV 846

The character of a piece is determined on the one hand by the composer's choice of variables, and on the other hand by the *rate of change of variables*. In our example, both the simplicity of the variables and their slow rate of change determine how the piece strikes us listeners: we hear a sense of evenness, of calm and simplicity, of easy flow. We understand readily how Charles Gounod was able to turn this prelude into a prayer (his 'Ave Maria').

Consciously or not, we observe the physical world as if it were a set of variables and constants. Doing so allows us to collect and analyze a great deal of information. We thus understand the nature of Bach's music, and that of Mozart, Beethoven, and everyone else.

Slowing Down the Rate of Change of Variables

The concept of variables and constants is extremely useful when you apply the Alexander Technique to solving technical and musical problems. It is a precise and comprehensive diagnostic tool. The difficulties of a passage or piece arise because a composer has chosen a large number of different variables; or because some of these variables are in themselves complex or out of the ordinary; or because the variables change too quickly for you to execute all of them cleanly and easily.

A solution arises quite logically out of such a diagnosis. In the first two cases, we simplify passages that contain a large number of variables, or we isolate complex variables and master them one by one; in both we establish *norms*, as discussed in Chapter 18, 'Norms and Deviations'. In the last case, in which variables change too quickly, we *slow down the rate of change of variables*. I explain.

In order to perform successfully any passage from your repertoire, you need to be comfortable with each variable contained in it and with the speed at which the variables change. Although sometimes the rate of change is uncomfortably slow, for most musicians technical difficulties arise when variables change too quickly.

Traditionally, musicians have dealt with such difficulties by practising the passages in question slowly. Useful as this may be, it is not always a true solution to the problem. When you play slowly a sequence of fast notes you use completely different mechanisms from the ones you use to play the sequence up to speed, just as you use your legs differently when you run and when you walk; walking is not the same as running slowly.

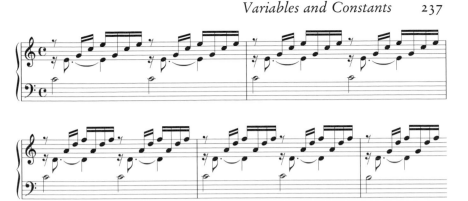

Ex. 20.2

Further, tempo and rhythm have a defining role in the character of a piece—more than, for instance, articulation or dynamics. To play a quick passage slowly will inevitably change the musical character of the passage, as well as its technical requirements. Technical mastery without musical mastery is not mastery at all.

Instead of practising slowly, keep intact those variables that determine the character of the piece and slow down not the passage's tempo but *its rate of change of variables*. I take Bach's prelude and play it as shown in Ex. 20.2. In Bach's original version there was one change of variable per bar. I have cut the rate of change in half, to one change of variable every two bars.

Breaking Down Automatic Responses

In Chapter 5, 'Direction', I discussed how Alexander developed a procedure for breaking down automatic reactions. (I suggest you reread the relevant section.) He had realized that every time he spoke he neglected to think up. His solution consisted in thinking up first and then alternating freely among three possible courses of action:

1. carrying on thinking up and doing nothing;
2. carrying on thinking up and doing something other than speaking (raising his hand, for instance);
3. carrying on thinking up and speaking.

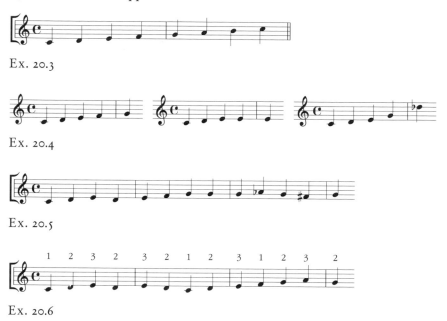

Ex. 20.3

Ex. 20.4

Ex. 20.5

Ex. 20.6

Soon he found that thinking up acquired enough pre-eminence and clarity in his mind for him to be able to think up and speak without difficulty.

In music-making, too, you always have the choice of doing what you are about to do, waiting a while before doing it, or doing something else altogether. Take the scale shown in Ex. 20.3. At any one point in the scale you have the choice of going ahead, of stopping at a certain note and repeating it, or simply playing any note you wish (see Ex. 20.4). You may also alternate freely, and execute the scale as shown in Ex. 20.5.

At the piano, to play a one-octave scale entails changing the position of the hand at least once. Let us say that I change the position of my hand once every four notes. (Other rates of change are also possible, depending on fingering.) If I change my one-octave scale into something like Ex. 20.6, I shall have slowed down the rate of change of variables. I no longer change hand positions after every four notes, but only after eight or more notes. This gives me more time to prepare each change—by inhibiting the desire to change too soon or too abruptly, by paying close attention to the pulse and to the rhythm of my movements, by thinking up along the spine, by directing the use of head, neck, and back as well as of my arm, hand, wrist, and fingers.

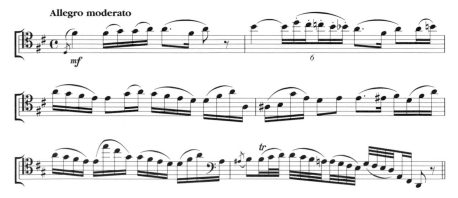

Ex. 20.7. From Joseph Haydn, Concerto in D major for cello and orchestra, Op. 101, first movement

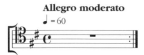

Ex. 20.8

An Illustration

I will proceed with a practical example before further explaining the procedure. Consider the opening solo phrase from Joseph Haydn's Concerto for cello and orchestra in D major, Op. 101 (Ex. 20.7). Cellists have long considered this a difficult piece which requires a great deal of virtuosity, as the many variables of rhythm, pitch, contour, figuration, left-hand positions, bow-strokes, bow-distribution, and articulation are difficult in themselves, and change at a nearly alarming rate.

The traditional solution to this problem consists of practising the passage slowly, carefully, grindingly. But as I said earlier, this so changes the character of the passage *and* its technical aspects that it cannot be considered a solution. Playing this passage slowly may even create difficulties anew.

Instead I keep intact the variables of pulse and musical character, so as to fulfil Haydn's intentions with every gesture of mine. I may choose to work with the metronome. I set it at sixty beats per minute, a good performing speed for this piece.

I start by *doing nothing*, a good working principle (see Ex. 20.8). I

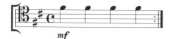

Ex. 20.9

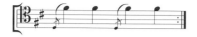

Ex. 20.10

organize my thoughts. First and foremost is my *thinking up along the spine*, which is not only a way of directing the head, neck, and back but an attitude as well. I make no assumptions about possible difficulties in front of me; I remain alert, confident, neither hesitant nor over-eager, ready to act and yet willing to wait. As I continue to think up, I check that the cello is well placed against my torso, that my legs are free from tension, that I am neither constricting nor forcing my breathing, that with my eyes I observe all around me with ease and with light-hearted detachment.

As I continue to think up (with all that it entails) I begin to plan the musical unfolding of the phrase ahead. I think of sound, full yet free; of articulation, clear and even; of forward motion, sure and compelling. I think of the work to be done by my arms, hands, and fingers. I hear the sounds of D major in my mind's ears. All of this I do while feeling without stop the steady pulse of Haydn's music even in silence.

Without losing my upward thought, and having prepared my gestures in the pulse and character of Haydn's lovely melody, I begin by playing a repeated note (Ex. 20.9). I have slowed down the rate of change considerably, but I have not eliminated those variables—tempo, pulse, articulation, bow-stroke—that, in the main, give the phrase its character. This simple, repeated note contains in it the seeds of the whole melody, and a listener may well have much pleasure in hearing me playing it. When I am assured of playing this note beautifully, in the spirit of Haydn and of Alexander, I add the little grace-note, not letting it disturb the steady, economical bow-stroke I established earlier (Ex. 20.10).

This task accomplished, I prepare to move on. Without ever stopping the repeated performance of my Haydn-like simple notes, I renew my upward and outward directions and move on to the next event in the melody (Ex. 20.11). Several variables change here: rhythm, articulation, bow-stroke, left-hand position. Yet I do not let any of

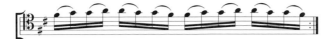

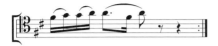

Ex. 20.11

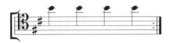

Ex. 20.12

Ex. 20.13

these changes disturb the musical flow I have established so far. I do not let the fear of changing left-hand positions make me move my left arm brusquely. Indeed, the rate of change of variables—my *psychological time*—is slow enough for me to have no fear altogether.

By repeating the first note many times, I have given myself plenty of time to prepare the new articulations and bow-strokes. I can then successfully prevent any unwanted accents or extraneous noises. I repeat this new figure enough times for me to become fully comfortable with it. Notice too that I alternate playing Haydn's original figure with its inversion. This may not appear in the original melody, but my execution of it is sufficiently Haydnesque not to detract from the character of the melody. When you search for freedom, more important than playing the right notes is for you to play each gesture with the right character, regardless of the notes. It is easy enough to find the right notes after you have cultivated a gesture's true nature; it is harder to instil character to right notes that you have learned with disregard for their musical nature.

Before long I decide I must not indulge for too long in the pleasurable sensations that this little pattern affords, and I move on (Ex. 20.12). This I handle with ease. I use the one-beat silence to renew my upward thought, which I never take for granted. My next task reminds me of the first note of the melody. I aim to play this note with the same bow-stroke and articulation that I had earlier (Ex. 20.13). This is not difficult to do. I find that I can play this note, continue to think up, and prepare the next gesture, which is somewhat trickier (Ex. 20.14).

Notice that although I have introduced one variable (the sextuplets

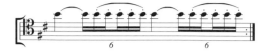

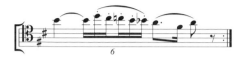

Ex. 20.14

Ex. 20.15

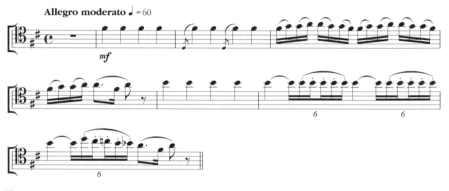

Ex. 20.16

and their attendant bow-stroke), I have delayed another (the sequence of descending pitches and their attendant left-hand activity). First I use my right hand with authority, then I bring this authority to bear upon my left hand. This we call the bilateral transfer, and we discussed it in Chapter 10, 'The Arms and Hands'. If my bow-strokes are clear, well-disciplined, light, and alive, and if I am satisfied that the upward thought animates my motions, I can then introduce the delightful figuration (Ex. 20.15).

Perhaps I need not illustrate the procedure any further. I apply the same principles of inhibition and direction, of discipline and improvisation, to the rest of the phrase.

Compare Haydn's original phrase with the way I practise it (Ex. 20.16). I maintain that, played with grace and control, this strange phrase is more Haydn-like, more to the point, more alive, and more useful than Haydn's original phrase played slowly, robotically, plod-dingly, as we hear it practised thousands of times by well-intended cellists all over the world. My transformation of Haydn's phrase is a marvellous way of learning how to think up and play at the same time. It helps me learn *inhibition in action*, as opposed to inhibition in waiting or in inaction. It helps me solve technical and musical problems without separating technical skill from musical content. And it offers me a gateway into the world of improvisation.

Improvisation

In the past improvisation was an integral part of every musician's daily life. To be a musician meant to be a composer, an improviser, and an interpreter. These activities were barely distinguishable from each other. No more; and undoubtedly this specialization of activities is a contributing factor to the shortcomings and ills of a modern musician.

Ask the average classical musician of today to improvise, for instance, a four-bar melody in the style of Mozart. His very first reaction is liable to be: 'No way!' He cannot, he will not, and he may even claim that he does not *want* to.

By definition, to improvise is to sing or play without knowing what is going to come out. To be afraid of improvising, then, is *to fear the unknown*. This universal fear always manifests itself in misuse of the whole self. To learn to improvise is to lose fear and, consequently, to stop misusing yourself.

I mentioned elsewhere that we all improvise when we speak. Free as it is, speech obeys certain strict rules of vocabulary and syntax. Musical improvisation, too, has its building-blocks and its syntax, but these are entirely outside the scope of this book.

From the Alexandrian point of view, to put playing the 'right notes' above all other considerations is to end-gain. To concentrate on the 'right notes' risks distracting you from the more important continuity of the musical line. Further, the continuity of the musical line is always allied to the continuity of a physical gesture. When one is continuous, so is the other; when one is disrupted, so is the other. Give up the 'right notes', slow down the rate of change of variables, improvise, and work on continuity of gesture and of music. You will then achieve all the freedom you need to play notes that are right, in letter and in spirit.

21 The Trampoline

Misuse of the Self and Technical Unreliability

Some aspects of music-making are common to a wide variety of musicians. String players, keyboard players, and trombonists, among others, all are faced with a particular problem: the need to make sudden, large, fast, and accurate arm gestures. A cellist, for instance, may need to change his left-hand position to cover the distance of an octave or more. A pianist's hand may have to travel from one limit of the keyboard to the other, sometimes over an extremely short time. And 'chromatic scales on the trombone', writes Denis Wick, 'present a problem which in a way sums up the main technical difficulties of the instrument—making long slide movements as effectively and as accurately as very short ones.'[1]

The Alexander Technique is ideally suited to handle this type of problem, as it provides an accurate diagnosis and a dependable remedy. Before we diagnose the problem, however, we need to describe it in greater detail.

Wick tells us what happens when a slide movement is badly executed: 'Young players often find that in a valiant effort to move the slide as quickly as possible they jerk it, so that the embouchure becomes disturbed—even battered—by the violence of the movement.'[2] The effect of the jerk on the embouchure is only part of a larger picture of misuse. Clearly the fast, vigorous movement of the arm disturbs the relationship of the head, neck, and back; it causes the head to be flung backwards and downwards, the neck to contract, the back to sway backwards, the pelvis to dip forwards. To compensate for a general loss of balance, the trombonist stiffens his legs, contracts his arms and shoulders, and constricts his breathing mechanisms.

Similar things happen to the cellist who makes a large shift with the left hand, or to the pianist whose hand leaps across the keyboard. Nearly every cellist shortens his spine and flings his head about with *each* change of position; the misuse is more exaggerated, and easier to observe, when the shifts are large, fast, or musically accented.

If a trombonist's embouchure is affected by a jerky arm movement, obviously his sound will suffer as well. Similarly, by contracting his spine with every left-hand shift the cellist of our example disturbs the continuity of his bow-line and ends up with a scratchy, uneven sound.

When a cellist or pianist misuses himself when making large, fast arm gestures, he is likely to miss his targeted note as well. There is little that frustrates a musician more than missing a note. The frustration of having missed, associated as it is with irritation, displeasure, and overeagerness, causes further failure, and soon a 'muscular memory of failure' grips the musician. Alexander wrote:

Every unsuccessful 'try' not only reinforces the pupil's old wrong psycho-physical habits associated with his conception of a particular act, but involves at the same time new emotional experiences of discouragement, worry, fear, and anxiety, so that the wrong experiences and the unduly excited reflex process involved in these experiences become one in the pupil's recognition; they 'make the meat they feed on.'[3]

Now we have a complete picture of misuse of the self. It includes the whole body, from head to toe; it is inextricably bound up with frustration in its many manifestations; and it affects every aspect of music-making.

Alexander wrote wryly that 'one would suppose that repeated experiences of failure would of itself lead [one] to set to work on a different principle'.[4] Yet if you take a walk down the corridors of a music college you will hear any number of students (and teachers) playing the same passage again and again, and missing the same notes every time. By doing so they are practising the problem, not its solution.

If the muscular memory of failure takes hold of you after you miss a note a few times, then your very wish to play the right note is likely to trigger a set reaction, characterized by the misuse of your self that causes you to miss the note. The solution is clear: you will need to abandon the strategy of executing the same faulty gesture repeatedly. Further, you will need to give up the very wish to get the right note, which is, in the last analysis, the reason why the gesture is faulty. Alexander wrote that a pupil must

learn by experience that *trying* to gain his end, *trying* to be right, is the surest way to failure.[5]

'Will-power' exerted by a pupil whose use of himself [is] misdirected would be exerted in the wrong direction. . . . It is not the degree of 'willing' or 'trying,' but the way in which the energy is directed, that is going to make the 'willing' or 'trying' effective.[6]

Paradoxical as it may seem, the pupil's only chance of success lies not in 'trying to be right,' but, on the contrary, in 'wanting to be wrong,' wrong, that is, according to any standard of his own.[7]

There are three separate phases to unlearning the faulty muscular memory of large, fast gestures. They involve cultivating a precise memory of the destination of the gesture; giving up the idea of hitting the right notes; and preparing the start of the gesture.

The Destination

Let your right arm hang by the side of your body. Now close your eyes and bring your right index finger up to your face quickly, and touch the tip of your nose. You are likely to miss your nose, or to hit it off centre, or to feel a little unsure of yourself even if you find your nose spot on.

Now tap your nose lightly but surely several times in rhythmic succession; let your arm hang by your side; and touch the tip of your nose again. I think you will find the target more easily, having acquired a precise muscular memory of the destination your hand reaches at the end of the gesture.

The pianist whose hands leap across the keyboard should use the same principle. Rather than practise the *journey* itself, he practises the *destination*, so that the journey may become easier. He plays the note or chord at the end of the gesture repeatedly, with great rhythmic clarity and drive, preferably in forte dynamics (as it makes the memory of the gesture clearer), always paying due attention to the use of his whole self: his head well poised at the end of his spine, his spine neither tight nor slack, his shoulders free, his back lengthening and widening, his legs participating fully and positively in the gesture. Working to this principle will guarantee that his memory of the desired end is clear, reliable, and imbued with freedom and confidence.

Being Wrong

As I pointed out earlier, you may need to dissociate a habitual misuse of your arm from the wish to find the right note that triggers the misuse. In other words, you need to lose your fear of missing notes. To do so, play wrong notes quite willingly, with confidence and pleasure.

Let us imagine that the passage you are practising demands a leap of one octave. Play the passage with all its required rhythmic flow, dynamics, and articulations, but allow yourself to miss the leap itself—play a ninth, a thirteenth, or any old note. You can let your hand fly right off the keyboard if you wish, as long as you do it with flair and with good use of your whole self. It is no good to miss a note and immediately correct it. As the cellist Christopher Bunting writes about correcting mistakes, 'the aim is not to acquire the skill of *"putting-things-right"* but of *"getting-things-right."*'[8]

In effect the point of this exercise is not to find the right note, but to move your arm without your habitual tensions. Give up getting the right note and you will find freedom; find freedom, and you will get the right note.

What characterizes a free arm in motion is not 'relaxation', but what we call *opposition*. This manifests itself in two different ways. First, there needs to be an opposition between the arm and the back, so that moving the arm does not disturb the head, neck, and back. For this to happen the spine must not be slack, or else the fast, vigorous arm motion will cause the head to contract into the neck in a whiplash-like effect.

Second, the gesture of the hand should be prepared by a slight movement (of the fingers, hand, or arm, according to the situation) away from the intended destination, not towards it. Watch a cat jump up on to a table, and you will see how she goes *down* before jumping *up*. This is a universal principle. The cellist who shifts his left hand from near the scroll to near the bridge (down in space but up in pitch) must point his arm in the direction opposite to the intended movement, as preparation for the movement itself. This helps release the arm and overcome the inertia of the hand position with a spring-like action.

The Trampoline

It is striking to an observant listener how the average musician prepares for important notes or notes difficult to play or sing: the moment before the big event there is a little hesitation, a little loss of

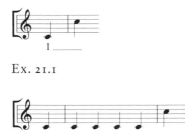

Ex. 21.1

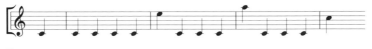

Ex. 21.2

Ex. 21.3

heart; musical attention falters and the continuity of the musical line is broken. This is a clear instance of end-gaining: the wish to get the high note (or to conquer whichever difficulty at hand) is such that the musician neglects the very means whereby the difficulty may be overcome.

'Caruso', wrote Viktor Fuchs, 'once mentioned in an interview in Berlin that the note before the high note is the most important.'[9] Play close attention to the preparation for the leap, and allow the leap itself to follow logically, naturally from all that precedes it. An athlete prepares a big jump on a trampoline by bouncing many times, thinking and yet not thinking of the jump that will surely come, readying himself by inhibiting the desire to jump prematurely. When he finally jumps, he shows the same certainty and vigour that he used in his preparatory bouncing.

In playing a leap at the keyboard, this involves 'thinking up', repeating the note (or chord) that precedes the leap several times in a row while respecting the pulse of the passage, and then proceeding with the leap while maintaining the confidence, good use, and rhythmic flow that you established on the repeated preparation note.

A cellist who needs to play the leap shown in Ex. 21.1 would then repeat the lower note until the conditions to leap were right (Ex. 21.2). Notice that you can combine this preparation with the idea of missing the high notes on purpose, and alternate long-delayed leaps onto the right notes with long-delayed leaps onto wrong notes: (Ex. 21.3). If this does not solve the problem, at least it will be a lot of fun.

22 *Imitation*

The Importance of Imitation

Human beings could not grow and learn, or even survive, if they did not possess remarkable innate powers of imitation. Imitation is present in every sphere of human activity, including all aspects of music-making. Although imitation is both necessary and inevitable, not all imitation is desirable. Two main questions arise: what to imitate, and how.

Let us look at the 'what' first, all the while keeping in mind that the 'how' always conditions the 'what' directly, and the 'what' conditions the 'how' indirectly. The first problem faced by every learner is the choice of models. All human beings are imperfect, therefore all models are in some way inadequate. This would not present a special problem if human beings today were not so pronouncedly imperfect. Thanks to the prevalence of end-gaining, the average modern man or woman is badly co-ordinated, unhealthy, unhappy, inadequate as a professional and as a person, doubly limited by birth and upbringing.

Circumstances usually predetermine the models you imitate. You do not choose your own parents, for instance, and you have to make do with whichever teachers you have at school. Circumstances apart, however, you risk making unwise choices, given several alternatives.

Once I had a colleague who was in awe of a famous cellist. Danny would go to every performance of his idol, score and pencil in hand, and would diligently write down as many fingerings and bowings as he could. He played the same pieces that his idol did, at the same speeds, with the same nuances. (We could say that he attempted to *execute* the *interpretations* of his idol.) He copied his idol's posture at the cello and his way of placing his instrument against his body. Danny would even copy the master's huffing and puffing, his facial expressions, the way he jutted his jaw forwards and tossed his head about.

Danny may have gone particularly far in his devotion, but he is in no way atypical of a young music student. His case illustrates many of the dangers associated with imitation. For us to appreciate how the Alexander Technique may help a musician avoid these dangers, we need to look at Danny's case in detail.

Artistry and Personality

First of all, let us consider Danny's choice of a model. An accomplished, successful musician does not automatically make a good model. Many musicians today achieve a measure of public success largely through the force of their personalities, rather than by means of technical and artistic mastery. 'Artistic judgement', wrote Wilhelm Furtwängler, 'has two sources, the thing itself, that is, the work of art, and "personality." The latter often has absolutely nothing to do with art and allows people to get away with all kinds of trickery.'[1]

Such musicians may well give their public great pleasure. And yet, however satisfying it may be to be taken in by a master trickster, once we examine his playing more closely we cannot fail to notice severe inadequacies of rhythm, technique, sound-production, articulation, style, and so on. The trickster succeeds despite his playing, not because of it. He emotes, he bluffs his way through performances, he *cheats*. But with such aplomb that he can get away with it.

The young musician who seeks inspiration in such a model misses an important point. His idol is successful thanks less to his artistry than to the force of his personality. The musician who imitates the individuality of another will never develop the force of his *own* personality. Therefore he will never become like his idol, whose defining characteristic is his *singularity*.

I made a similar point in Chapter 16, 'Daily Practice', when I wrote about a violinist who practises ceaselessly in the hope of being 'like Heifetz'. Heifetz himself practised sparingly and intelligently. The best way to be 'like Heifetz', and to pay him homage, is to emulate the intelligence of his working methods. These allowed him to fulfil his own potential, and may help you to fulfil yours.

Interpretation, Authority, and Fallibility

Danny copies his idol's bowings and fingerings. This fails to take two points into account. First, bowings and fingerings, as well as all other elements of a musician's execution, ought to have a certain inner logic. They must serve the needs of the music, they are bound somewhat by the physical characteristics of the instrument, and they must conform to the morphology and the use of the individual musician. Hand size and the stretch between individual fingers, for instance, sometimes restrict the choice of fingerings. It seems unlikely that Danny will understand the logic of his idol's choices by imitating them. Further, these choices may possibly be suited to the idol himself, but not to the fan.

Second, great musicians are not infallible. They make unintelligent choices from time to time; some successful artists make *consistently* stupid choices. Musical editions prepared and signed by well-known musicians come with all sorts of indications: bowings, fingerings, breathing and articulation marks, pedalling, and many others. It is both amusing and appalling to see how haphazard and inadequate these indications can be. To imitate the mistakes of others is not a good idea. You have all the right in the world to make your own mistakes, particularly if in the process you learn the laws of fingering, bowing, breathing, and so on.

Worse still is to assign automatic musical authority to a musician who is well known. A chamber music coach once suggested a tempo for a movement my string quartet was studying. I asked him to explain his choice, which was bewildering to me. He replied, 'The Juilliard Quartet play so.' The Juilliard are a great group indeed. Does that mean they never get it wrong, or that their choices, when right, preclude all other choices? Definitely not. And even if I end up choosing exactly the same tempo as the Juilliard, I should do so not by parrot-like imitation but thanks to an artistic understanding of the reasons behind their choices.

Copying Defects

Besides copying some outward signs of his idol's technique, Danny copies many of his mannerisms, which are in no way necessary to the artistic rendition of a piece. Alexander was fond of saying that an artist succeeds despite his faults, not because of them. Danny will not become a better cellist by copying someone else's defects; quite the contrary.

A sense of proportion and balance is inherent in the ideal of human perfection. Every exaggeration is by definition a defect; in a well-co-ordinated person nothing is excessive, nothing is out of place. Yet exaggerated peculiarities are more easily noticed, and therefore more readily imitated, than the subtleties of moderate behaviour. A good model may go unnoticed precisely because of his goodness. Presented with such a model, the person of average misuse (and average sensory misapprehension) may either not know that he is indeed facing a good model, or know that the model is good, but not how or why.

An observer who faces a good model, and who is willing to copy some of this model's worthy characteristics, still runs into two ever-present difficulties. Thanks to faulty sensory awareness, you may think (or, more precisely, feel) that you are copying the model as he is, when in effect you are copying him as you perceive him to be. If there are ten students in an exercise or dance class, there will be ten different ways of imitating the teacher, and most of these will be useless or even harmful to the student.

Misuse and Imitation

Let us now imagine that you choose a good model, and that you make a precise assessment of what you must imitate. You still face what is perhaps the greatest difficulty in imitation: your being able to actually imitate what you see. Take a look at the photograph of George Balanchine and Arthur Mitchell in Chapter 5, 'Direction'. In all likelihood, Mitchell is trying to imitate Balanchine. Indeed, we can suppose that he is trying to do exactly as Balanchine does, and that he believes that he is doing so. Yet there are several remarkable differences between the two men. Can you spot them? Do you think that, as he dances, Mitchell himself is aware of these differences? How easily do you think that Mitchell could make changes in his use, the better to imitate Balanchine? Could Balanchine imitate Mitchell more easily? Perhaps after looking at this photo you decide that you prefer Mitchell's style of dancing to Balanchine's. Can you come up with some arguments other than 'I just like him better' to justify your preference?

Before we proceed any further, let us draw a first set of conclusions about imitation.

1. Everybody has an innate ability to imitate. We need this ability to survive, to learn, to grow. We exercise our powers of imitation both consciously and subconsciously.
2. Imitation can be a power for good or for bad, depending on whom we imitate and why and how.
3. The prevalence of end-gaining and misuse makes it difficult to find good models.
4. We tend not to appreciate good models when in their presence; our attention is more easily caught by exaggerated characteristics, which are defects by definition.
5. Prominent or successful men and women are not necessarily good models. Prominence does not equal authority, and authority does not equal infallibility.
6. Models are never wholly good; a model may be good despite his faults, and we must be able to distinguish a model's defects from his good qualities, and copy only the latter.
7. Because of faulty sensory awareness we tend to imitate even a good model incorrectly.

Models of Good Use

'A great singer', wrote Husler and Rodd-Marling, 'can always imitate the poor tones of a non-singer—either by omitting to use certain parts of his vocal organ or by disturbing its proper physiological functioning.'[2] The great singer is in command of his own use, and can therefore produce all that he wishes with his voice, including dozens of imitations and caricatures of other singers. But could the lesser singer imitate the greater one? Not before he acquires the same mastery of his use.

We have reached the crux of the matter. For imitation to be operative and healthy, we must imitate not effects but causes, not the outward manifestations of co-ordination but the co-ordinative processes themselves, not the *functioning* of the self but its *use*.

The observer who looks at the world in an Alexandrian frame of mind is struck by remarkable similarities between profoundly different human beings. Artur Rubinstein, Jascha Heifetz, William Primrose, and Emanuel Feuermann (pianist, violinist, violist, and cellist respectively) all expressed their artistry in ways unique to each of them. And yet there was so much in common to all of them: their composure, their economy of means, their focused energy, their complete mastery of their instruments, their magnetism on stage—in sum, their artistic outlook and the means they used to actualize it.

In performance, they were neither too tense nor too slack. They moved their bodies with discretion and elegance, always keeping the relationship between their head, neck, and back constant, dynamic, organic but not fixed. The energy they had at their fingertips arose from their powerful, solid backs, and it travelled through arms and wrists that were poised and ready for work, neither floppy nor tightened. Their features revealed utter involvement with their music-making and a certain detachment as well; they created enormous excitement in the audience without being themselves overrun by excitement. They were and remain extremely good models—not because they were striking or endearing, nor because they were prominent, but simply because they used themselves well.

Personal likes and dislikes need not come into play in Alexandrian imitation. You do not have to agree with Heifetz's interpretations or approve of the way he treated his wives in order to adopt him as one of your models. In Chapter 17, 'Aesthetic Judgements', I discussed the difference between standards of right and wrong that are absolute and immutable, and standards of right and wrong that vary according to circumstance. Heifetz's stylistic choices were perhaps right at his time, less so today; but his use at the violin was *intrinsically* right and will remain so for ever.

I pointed out earlier how it is impossible for you to affirm your own individuality by copying someone else's singularity. Paradoxical as it may seem, it is by copying what is *universal* in a model that you take the first step in affirming your individuality.

Rubinstein, Heifetz, Primrose, and Feuermann all have highly individual voices, despite everything that makes them similar to one another. If we compare not players of different instruments but different players of the same instrument, we see greatness again as the individual flowering of universal principles. The pianists Vlado Perlemuter, Jorge Bolet, Nikita Magaloff, Shura Cherkassy, and Lili Kraus, to mention just a few, all share several characteristics of use. Yet there would be no mistaking the playing of one for the playing of another. It is clear that you can imitate their common use and not only retain your individuality but enhance it.

The Alexander Technique and Imitation

Let us draw a second set of conclusions about imitation, now highlighting the ways in which the Alexander Technique makes imitation effective and beneficial.

1. The Alexander Technique provides clear, objective, definable, consistent criteria for the use of the self, thereby allowing you as an observer to determine what a good model is.
2. A good model is a person who uses himself well. Imitate his use, not his functioning.
3. To imitate others well, you need to *see* both yourself and the world around you clearly, and to use yourself well enough to translate something you *see* into something you *do*.

Keeping in mind all of the preceding observations, let us now consider what you can do to imitate good models in a constructive manner.

1. Seek to be in the presence of people with good use. When in the presence of people with bad use, be sure *not* to lose your own upward orientation. Once you become aware of use—your own and others'—you will be surprised at how prevalent imitation is, and how readily everybody imitates a person with bad use and a strong personality. This is clear in the case of children and their parents, for instance. I once saw a tall man stoop to pass under a low door-frame; his three-year-old watched him and also stooped as he went along.

2. Watch concerts, films, and videos with a constant awareness of the use of the performers. Find out about performers whose use is good and make a conscientious effort to go to their concerts and collect their videos.

3. Develop an appreciation of what is good in an imperfect model, and copy it accordingly. One of my cello teachers never practised the cello or performed the solo literature; he was often 'out of form'. Yet when he gave demonstrations at the cello he always had such a positive upward and outward orientation of his whole being that I always benefited from imitating him, even when he played out of tune and with a scratchy sound. I imitated his use, not his playing.

4. Because the vast majority of people misuse themselves most of the time, to observe others with Alexandrian eyes is to observe misuse. This is an education in what *not* to do; if you are aware of the

mechanics of imitation, you can consciously fashion yourself after a good model and after the *opposite* of a bad one if need be. Two pupils of mine, Nathalie and Olivier, once shared a lesson. I was giving Olivier a turn, and I had run into some resistance from Olivier over a particular procedure I wanted to lead him through. Up to then Nathalie had always presented the same resistance in her private lessons. Suddenly, she grasped the nature of her previous behaviour—by seeing somebody else behave in the same way. She had a strong, practical reaction to seeing a wrong model: she knew she would rather be unlike what she saw, and she did not offer any resistance when her turn came.

5. If you are going to imitate universal aspects of good use, then you do not have to limit your models to people who are in your field of activity. A cellist may draw inspiration from a pianist, a pianist from a dancer, a dancer from a potter, a man from a woman, an adult from a child. I would like to play the cello as well as Art Blakey plays the drums; I learn more about how to become a good cellist from watching Blakey than I do from watching an experienced cellist with bad use.

6. You are better off copying an inexperienced model who uses himself well than an accomplished one who uses himself badly. When I first took up ice-skating, I watched closely a four-year-old child who was just beginning to skate, and who was a paragon of good use. There were some older boys who whizzed confidently by, their bodies contracted and distorted by the overeagerness of end-gaining. Although the little boy went carefully and slowly around the rink, he was a better teacher, for me and everybody else, than the faster, cocksure kids.

7. I have written so far of you imitating others. All my observations apply equally to others imitating you. Inevitably some people will indeed copy you, whether or not they (or you) are aware of it.

'Could any fault weigh heavier on a human conscience', cautions Alexander, 'than that by which, however unwittingly, another human life had been distorted?'[3] I believe that we all should strive to be good models for others. We often attempt to influence others directly: by force, manipulation and blackmail, by nagging, pleading, hectoring, commanding. To change yourself is infinitely better than to change others, and to be a living model of good use is perhaps the best way of indirectly helping others.

23 Stage Fright

The Causes of Stage Fright

Remember Alexander's words on the nature of his work: 'You are not here to do exercises, or to learn to do something right, but to get able to meet a stimulus that always puts you wrong and to learn to deal with it.'[1] Stage fright merits two approaches. The first is to learn its causes and find a permanent remedy for it. The second is to consider it 'a stimulus' that 'puts you wrong', and 'learn to deal with it': that is, perform successfully despite stage fright. I believe the Alexander Technique offers all musicians effective ways of eliminating stage fright *and* of dealing with it when it is there. Before we read what Alexander has to say about stage fright, let us consider some of its more immediate causes.

1. *Technical and musical insufficiency*. A musician whose technique and musicianship are inadequate to the task at hand may well suffer from stage fright. Perhaps he has chosen too difficult a piece, or has not given it adequate preparation. Let us call this *warranted* stage fright. It is only natural to be afraid of performing, in exceptional circumstances, something you cannot play in *normal* circumstances. (On rare occasions, exceptional circumstances lead people to overcome their inadequacies as if by miracle, but it would be foolish for an unprepared performer to count on this happening.) Before a musician can give some thought to stage fright as such, he needs first to acquire sufficient skill and polish. This is not to say that only accomplished performers ought to go on stage; obviously every musician has to go through an apprenticeship that entails performing as an inexperienced beginner. My argument about insufficient or inadequate preparation as a source of stage fright applies equally to a concert artist playing a major work and to a beginner playing a simple piece.

2. *Stupidity in living*. Stage fright sometimes comes about if a musician, well prepared though he may be technically and musically,

neglects some of the aspects of concert preparation that are not directly related to music-making. A night badly slept, a heavy meal, the intake of alcohol and coffee, arriving late to the concert-hall, can all hinder a musician's ability to focus on the performance. Heinrich Neuhaus wrote:

When, after a concert or a number of concerts, I sometimes considered why the concert was as it was and not different, I could very easily establish a connection between the quality of the concert and the mode of life that preceded it. . . . ([Alfred] Cortot used to say that for a concert pianist on tour the most important thing is sound sleep and a good digestion.)[2]

Good sense dictates a number of rules regarding the daily life of a performing artist. Not to follow them is simply unintelligent, and the Alexander Technique goes only so far in compensating for stupidity. (Interestingly enough, the long-term study of the Alexander Technique may lead to many changes in lifestyle. Drinking, smoking, or eating heavily may cause you to lose your upward and outward orientation. In time you will come to prefer *being up* to *being down*, and you will lose the desire to indulge yourself.)

3. *Unusual circumstances.* Sometimes one or more details in the circumstances of the concert may trigger stage fright in a musician who is thoroughly well prepared, sober, well fed, and well rested. There is a delay of a few minutes before the start of the concert; the stage lighting is different from the rehearsal; there is a draught; the floor squeaks; a child coughs in the third row. In reality circumstances are almost never ideal. True professionals take account of imperfections in the settings of their performances, and either are not bothered by them or play well despite being bothered. This attitude is also an artistic outlook: The music I am playing is truly great; from it I derive boundless inspiration; my audience will be enraptured even if a cat chases a mouse under the piano. To deal with stage fright in these circumstances you need both to cultivate the necessary artistic outlook, and to submit yourself in daily practice willingly, with conscientious discipline, to the stimuli of abnormal circumstances. This I discussed in Chapter 14, 'Working on Yourself'. There I argued that the problem lies not in the stimuli of unusual circumstances, but in your reaction to them. Learn to inhibit all interference to your Primary Control, and you need not fear the unexpected or the abnormal. We shall come back to this shortly.

The Alexandrian Framework

We have so far considered cases of stage fright caused by technical and musical insufficiency, by lack of common sense in the run-up to a performance, and by startling or annoying details in the circumstances of the concert. It is relatively easy to solve or mitigate stage fright thus caused. More intriguing is the stage fright that strikes a well-prepared, accomplished musician who plays in unexceptional circumstances.

We find in Alexander's writings a statement of the causes of stage fright, its manifestations, and its remedy. He wrote:

We are told that [stage fright] is all a matter of 'nerves' and so forth. . . . These emotional disturbances [are] part and parcel of an unbalanced psycho-physical condition, of a state of anxiety and confusion, and there can be little doubt that any circumstance that is more or less unusual is likely to bring about a recurrence of the same disturbed psycho-physical condition.[3]

Elsewhere Alexander discussed professional athletes who suffer from stage fright and perform badly in big events:

It is probable that anyone with a knowledge of what constitutes interference with the primary control of use would be able to observe in these players such varying interference with this control as could account for the variation in the standard of their play at different times. The manner of interference varies with the different ways of using the self, and the degree of interference tends to increase with repetition.[4]

I have long been a fan of Steve Cram, the great British middle-distance runner. At his best—when he broke the mile record in 1984, for instance—his use was exemplary. His whole being was oriented upwards and outwards; his energies were collected, his motions economical, his strides powerful. His use being so good when he was on form, it was all the more educational to observe him when he was off form. The relationship between his head, neck, and back deteriorated visibly. His head would bob sideways and backwards and forwards. His whole co-ordination suffered as a result, and so did his ability to win a race. He illustrated to perfection the relationship between use and performance in high-pressure situations.

As to the remedy to stage fright, Alexander wrote that in a lesson the teacher asks his pupil not to make any attempt to gain the 'end' at all, but instead to learn gradually to remember the guiding orders or directions, which are the forerunners of the *means whereby* the end may one day be gained. This may not be today, tomorrow or the next day, but it will be, and then the pupils will be able to repeat the act with mathematical precision at all times and under all circumstances, for such retarding factors as unduly excited fear reflexes, uncontrolled emotions and fixed prejudices will not have been developed in the process just outlined.

... The relation of all this to the very important question of the ability to 'keep one's head' at critical moments is clear.[5]

Stage fright, then, is but a symptom of an 'unbalanced disturbed psychophysical condition', a symptom of the *misuse of the self*. It is characterized by *interference with the Primary Control*, and its remedy is the *inhibition* of the *end-gaining* that causes it, and the *direction* of the *means whereby* any end may be achieved.

The soundness of Alexander's approach is evident in three ways. First, Alexander does not speak of 'physical', 'mental', or 'social' causes of stage fright. By considering the individual whole Alexander does him the greater service. Second, he sees stage fright as a specific manifestation of a general phenomenon. By working on the use of the *whole* self, on a *general* basis, and allowing functioning (of which stage fright, or its absence, is but one aspect in many) to improve *indirectly*, we achieve in one swoop multiple results that are comprehensive, solid, and long-lasting. Third, Alexander sees the solution to stage fright not as a *doing*, but a *non-doing*—preventing the misuse of the Primary Control. The merits of *not* doing something to combat stage fright directly may not be evident at first, yet most musicians are familiar with the increase in stage fright that comes with wilful efforts to control it.

The procedures outlined in this book all follow Alexander's framework of end-gaining, misuse, inhibition, and direction. Apply them steadily in your daily work, and you may well lose your fear of stage fright. I repeat Alexander's words: 'This may not be today, tomorrow or the next day, but it will be.'

The aim is to rid yourself of the very notion of stage fright. An actor before he was a teacher, Alexander used to direct his own pupils and trainees in plays that were performed publicly. Writing about one of these productions, he said that because his students had prepared their performances along the principles of his Technique, 'the idea of "stage fright" was one that seemed to them the merest absurdity. It may be said that they did not understand what was meant by such a condition.'[6]

Emotions and Bodily Reactions

I should like to highlight and clarify one aspect of Alexander's understanding, namely the inseparability of body and mind. William James, generally considered the father of modern psychology, wrote in his *Textbook of Psychology*:

Our natural way of thinking about these coarser emotions (e.g. 'grief, fear, rage, love') is that the mental perception of some fact excites the mental affection called the emotion, and that this latter state of mind gives rise to the bodily expression. My theory, on the contrary, is that *the bodily changes follow directly from the perception of the exciting fact and that our feeling of the same changes as they occur* IS *the emotion.... Every one of the bodily changes, whatsoever it be, is* FELT *acutely or obscurely, the moment it occurs.* If the reader has never paid attention to this matter, he will be both interested and astonished to learn how many different local bodily feelings he can detect in himself as characteristic of his various emotional moods.... If we fancy some strong emotions and then try to abstract from our consciousness of it all the feelings of its bodily symptoms we find we have nothing left behind, no 'mind-stuff' out of which the emotion can be constituted, and that a cold and neutral state of intellectual perception is all that remains.[7]

This idea runs counter to common assumptions about the relationship between body and mind. We believe that we apprehend fear of failure, for instance, in our minds; that this apprehension 'gives' us stage fright; and that stage fright in turn causes our limbs to shake and our breathing and digestion to become abnormal. By proposing that a mental perception precedes a bodily state and causes it, this subtly implies a separation between body and mind. James suggests that the bodily state *is* the emotion. Interestingly, modern science is now validating James's century-old view. Current neurobiological research argues that 'emotions and feelings are not, as poets and philosophers say, ephemeral reflections of the human soul', but rather 'the brain's interpretation of our visceral reaction to the world at large'.[8]

Perhaps you remember Alexander's quote about the 'subconsciousness': his conception of it 'does not necessarily imply any distinction between the thing controlled and the control itself'.[9] The mind does not control the body; the body does not control the mind. There are no 'states of mind' or 'states of body', only *states of self*. Stage fright is one such state, and when dealing with it you must not lose sight of Alexander's, and James's, fundamental insight.

The Condition of Stage Fright

We tend to speak of stage fright as if we all agreed on what we mean by the expression—as if stage fright were a single phenomenon, experienced by all in the same light. Maria Callas and Pablo Casals, among many other great artists, suffered from stage fright all their lives, yet their every performance was thrilling to the audience and, surely at least on some occasions, to themselves. Tito Gobbi, who sang frequently with Callas, recounts amusingly:

Despite [Callas's] tremendous, unparalleled triumph she remained desperately nervous. On each day of performance she would phone me to say she could not sing—she had no voice left, or else she must change everything in the second act. I would be half-an-hour on the telephone consoling the poor girl and encouraging her. 'All right,' I would say, 'you don't sing. It is enough for you to appear. You just act and I'll do the singing—All right, you change whatever you want. You know we understand each other—,' and so on.[10]

Stage fright is but a reaction to a stimulus. The stimulus may be universal to all performers, but the reaction to it varies from person to person. Callas responded to stage fright in a way that, uncomfortable as it may have been, effectively enhanced her performances. She excelled because of her stage fright, not despite it. Bruce Lee wrote that 'the experienced athlete recognizes [the presence of stage fright] *not as an inner weakness*, but as *an inner surplus*'.[11] I suspect that, offered a choice, Callas would not have given up her stage fright if that entailed giving lacklustre performances.

To a lucky few, the anticipation of a performance and the performance itself are both wholly positive. To others (like Callas and Casals), the anticipation is negative, yet the performance positive. To others yet, both anticipation and actual performance are negative. Further, these negative reactions manifest themselves differently in different musicians. Some shake, others have the 'runs', other still have an urge to fall asleep.

In sum, stage fright means different things to different performers. It manifests itself in ways unique to each individual and it may even be a positive phenomenon, a way for a performer to force herself to heights greater than she would achieve in the absence of stage fright.

We have so far examined different types of stage fright and their possible causes and remedies. We have also looked at the Alexandrian framework, which provides long-term, indirect procedures of eliminating stage fright. We can now consider short-term, direct strategies for dealing with it, although precisely because they are short-term and direct they cannot take the place of the true 'means whereby' stage fright is eliminated. There are four different aspects to be considered: inner preparation, the anticipation of stage fright, the use of rituals, and green-room conduct.

Inner Preparation

By 'inner preparation' I mean the psycho-physical exercises in imagination and visualization that allow you to *conceive* of yourself as an accomplished performer before you become one. In Chapter 5, 'Direction', I made the point that visualization is not synonymous with direction. Alexander himself sounded a cautionary note against visualization: 'If a person whose sensory awareness is untrustworthy places reliance upon a picture he "visualizes" or a feeling he "senses," he is depending . . . on an illusory basis of rightness. Unless some provision can be made for changing and improving this condition of unreliable sensory appreciation . . . , in what way can these procedures be of benefit to him?'[12]

A badly co-ordinated person risks disco-ordinating himself further by visualizing. By the same measure, however, the well-co-ordinated person risks nothing by visualizing, and may well gain from it. Most of the leading athletes of today make extensive use of their powers of visualization to prepare for competition. If you direct your whole self before and during visualization, then you too can use it to improve your performances.

I shall not go into visualization in detail, as this would be outside the scope of this book. Rather, I would like to suggest some ways in which the Alexander Technique may be used in conjunction with it.

Place yourself in a position of mechanical advantage (the monkey, the lunge, or semi-supine, for instance). Send upward and outward directions for your whole self. Then carry on with these directions as you visualize, thereby creating a connection between your good use and the images of successful performance. You may use all the common techniques for visualizing: imagine yourself performing, imagine yourself as a member of the audience watching you perform, imagine the audience's pleasure in your performance.

Anticipating Stage Fright

Traditionally musicians have used visualization to imagine themselves free from stage fright. Another route is also possible.

Place yourself in a position of mechanical advantage, or pace the room, sit, or stand as you wish. Give your directions. Then imagine yourself in a concert situation, *suffering from stage fright*. This is very easily done. I think you will soon feel your habitual symptoms of stage fright: queasiness, shaking, and so on. Carry on visualizing, and renew your upward and outward directions. Think of the elasticity of your spine and the strength in your back and legs, the looseness of your jaw and tongue, the natural expansion of your ribcage as you breathe. In other words, 'think up' even as you suffer from the effects of stage fright.

Do this deliberately and conscientiously. Time it well in advance of a performance. Do it every day for a while. This exercise is painful, and you may need to force yourself to go through it. Yet the rewards of the discipline justify the effort. Two things may well happen. First, your upward and outward directions slowly become more present and powerful than your imagined stage fright, and end by overcoming it. Second, by the time the concert occasion arrives, you will have spent all your capacity for fearing stage fright and worrying about it. Alexander wrote about the 'worry habit, a state in which [a person] manufactures the stimulus to worry.'[13] I do not suggest that you cultivate this nasty habit, but rather that you find ways of letting your good use supplant it.

On Rituals, Superstition, and Concentration

'The great challenge in performing in public', wrote the pianist Gyorgy Sandor, 'comes from the way the environment of a live concert differs from your practice room.'[14] The practice room is ordinary, the concert stage extraordinary. The extraordinariness of performance is twofold. You can practise as much and as often as you like, but in all likelihood you will not have the opportunity to perform as much and as often as you practise. Performing is extraordinary because less frequent than practising. But it remains extraordinary even when it does become frequent. The concert artist who plays a hundred or more recitals a year still finds that walking on stage is not to be likened to any other experience. Performing is extraordinary because it is exalted. To perform frequently, useful as it is, does not automatically eliminate stage fright, as it does not change the exalted nature of performance.

You respond to the exaltation of a concert situation by entering an extraordinary state of self. To better deal with this state, you can trigger it away from the stage by using pre-concert rituals.

Each musician has a personal ritual of choice: ironing a blouse, shining a pair of concert shoes, showering or applying make-up, going for a quiet walk or praying. To prescribe a ritual for everyone would be counter-productive, but a few guidelines may be useful.

It is important to distinguish between rituals that concentrate the mind and that are wholly beneficial, and rituals that are superstitious in nature and that possibly create the risk of greater stage fright. Useful rituals help the purposes of self-discipline, of finding the inner strength to respond to an extraordinary situation. Superstition, on the other hand ('If I wear my polka dot underwear, nothing can go wrong'), is an escape from the risks and responsibilities that you face when you go on stage, and it is based on wishful thinking rather than inhibiting and directing. It can also go terribly wrong. What if the polka dot underwear is in the wash? Ultimately it is the purpose of the ritual that makes it positive, not its form.

Another important aspect of positive ritual is that it should not address your frame of mind alone but the use of your whole self. Alexander wrote emphatically about 'mind wandering' and concentration. He argued that mind wandering is a condition of the whole psychophysical being, and that concentration as ordinarily understood and practised is as undesirable as the condition it is meant to remedy. I wrote about the distinction between concentration and awareness in Chapter 5, 'Direction'. I repeat two quotes from Bruce Lee: 'classical concentration . . . focuses on one thing and excludes all others, and awareness . . . is total and excludes nothing.'[15] 'A concentrated mind is not an attentive mind but a mind that is in the state of awareness can concentrate.'[16]

Many musicians have tried to combat stage fright by 'concentrating', and have used rituals with this purpose. Rituals should be primarily a process of addition, not subtraction. Rather than trying to exclude the apparent distractions that 'take your mind away' from the task at hand, it is more beneficial to *add* the awareness of your head, neck, back, and whole organism to the activities that precede a concert. You may feel strongly that to think of your neck may distract you from your playing and make you play worse. Yet the better you use yourself, the better you will play. I hope you have accepted this as axiomatic by now. Use pre-concert rituals, then, not to concentrate on your performing, but rather to acquire a heightened awareness of your use, which will help your performing as surely as day follows night.

In the Green-Room

The green-room gets its name from the unlovely hue of every performer's face before he goes on stage. Most of the strategies I have outlined so far are meant for the long and medium term. By the time you get to the green-room it may be too late to save the day. Nevertheless, you can and should use the Alexander Technique up to the very moment you step on stage and beyond.

First we must consider yet again the issue of tension and relaxation. Many musicians believe that stage fright is caused by too much tension, and that its solution is relaxation. This is a misunderstanding of the nature of tension and its role in performance. 'Tension', I argued in Chapter 1, 'creates and sustains life, and carries it forwards. Tension—of the right kind—is a prerequisite of dynamic, energetic, vital human endeavour.' Tension is inevitable, necessary, and desirable. A well-co-ordinated performer is not relaxed but *collected*: 'possessed of calmness and composure often through concentrated effort' (*Webster's Ninth New Collegiate Dictionary*). 'Collected' has a second meaning, 'gathered together', which also applies in this case. What a performer needs, then, is not to eliminate tension but to direct and harness it, and make it serve its proper artistic purpose.

Sometimes the harnessing of tension will not happen in a calm and composed manner. Heinrich Neuhaus recounts an instructive anecdote about the great nineteenth-century pianist Anton Rubinstein (not a relation of Artur), who 'was very nervous and once even broke a mirror in the artist's room with his fist before walking on to the platform (this seemed to have calmed him)'.[17] Punching a mirror is perhaps too injurious a solution, but it is more true to the nature of artistic tension than the relaxation and deep breathing exercises usually prescribed for pre-concert nerves. I do not recommend it; instead, I suggest a series of lively and vigorous monkeys, lunges, and whispered 'ah's, the purpose of which is not to relax you but to awaken and direct the various tensions necessary for performance.

A word about the whispered 'ah'. As I insisted when I first discussed it, it is not a breathing exercise but a co-ordinative procedure, and it affects breathing but indirectly. For your whispered 'ah's to be useful in the green-room, you need to give up the very idea of controlling breathing, or of using breathing to control your emotions. The one thing you can influence directly is the working of your Primary Control—the relationship between head, neck, and back. And even then there is not much for you to *do*; instead you must *undo* or *not do*, as the case may be. This surely is the answer to stage fright, as it is to most other problems.

On Confidence

There are men and women who, despite great inadequacies of character and ability, are supremely assured of themselves. This unwarranted self-assurance, a delusion of sorts, has served some people well but ruined many others, and cannot be considered in any way desirable.

Its contrary, a profound insecurity that paralyses otherwise able men and women, is no more desirable. 'Too modest is half-proud', says a Jewish proverb. Successful performers, or, more broadly, successful human beings who perform successfully, eschew both the empty self-assurance engendered by positive thinking and the undue modesty that passes for humility. '*Vanity and confidence*', wrote Wilhelm Furtwängler, '. . . sometimes look as alike as twins. And yet no two things could be more different. One is the necessary accompaniment of all great achievement, the other a burden.'[18]

Daily practice and daily life both should contribute, steadily and unfailingly, to an improvement in your use, and to a consequent increase in confidence. 'The healthy person needs a certain arrogance,'

Furtwängler wrote; 'nature has made sure of that.'[19] Use yourself well, and be glad of your good use; then bring both your good use and your healthy pride in it to your performances.

On Beta-Blockers

Beta-blockers are a relatively new class of drugs. Originally meant for the treatment of angina and high blood pressure, they were soon being used by performers and athletes for the suppression of stage fright and the enhancement of their performances. (In some sports their use has since been declared illegal.)

Many musicians have found beta-blockers extremely effective in dealing with stage fright. Some claim that, unlike tranquillizers, beta-blockers do not turn them into unexcited or unexciting performers; rather, they allow for the excitement of a performance without the crippling effects of stage fright. It may be fair to say that beta-blockers have saved the careers of some musicians. Does the success of beta-blockers contradict the Alexander Technique in any way?

We must note that beta-blockers, powerful drugs that they are, may have serious side-effects, including 'lethargy, constriction of the smaller air-passages, aggravation of asthma, spasm of arteries in the legs to worsen pain on walking (claudication), and even, though rarely, spasm of the coronary arteries to worsen the very angina that the drug was supposed to prevent',[20] as well as a diminution of sexual appetite. Clearly, in the long term beta-blockers may be more a problem than a solution.

Yet, as I noted earlier, to build up your confidence as a performer it is not enough to perform frequently. If you give five failed performances in a row, you may well expect to fail the sixth time around—and you risk failing as the result of a self-fulfilling prophecy, a vicious circle which may be difficult to break.

I believe that the use of beta-blockers may be justified for two purposes (but *never* positively recommended): to combat crippling stage fright before you have acquired sufficient knowledge of the Alexander Technique, and to break the vicious circle of failure. If you do decide to take beta-blockers (and I sincerely hope that you find other, better ways of handling stage fright), then make the best of it and bring an awareness of your use to your drug-aided performance, so that you begin to associate good use and success. Eventually good use itself becomes the *source* of success, not one of its characteristics. If, however, you neglect to draw this lesson from performances for which you have taken beta-blockers, you will endanger both your health and your career.

Every doctor is a fool; we all know that. But a greater fool is he who takes drugs without the supervision of an able and sympathetic doctor. Keep in mind that beta-blockers are powerful and potentially harmful drugs, and do not misuse or abuse them. Be willing, too, to explore homeopathic alternatives such as gelsemium.

A Negation of Alexander's View

Earlier I discussed the way Alexander viewed stage fright. For him, performers who do not end-gain would consider stage fright 'the merest absurdity', and would 'not understand what was meant by such a condition.' I am sure many of my readers would dearly wish to 'not understand' what is meant by stage fright, and never to experience it. To consider stage fright an absurdity, something unimaginable, is a view of the nature of performance that I cherish. Yet I also appreciate the contrary view, expressed poignantly and convincingly by Heinrich Neuhaus:

Such nervousness as that of [Anton] Rubinstein is, I think, due partly to the fact that every public performance is subject to 'the power of the moment' and the highly artistic personality capable of inspiration is more liable to be affected by it than the standard, balanced artists who experience neither great flights nor great falls. . . . But the main reason is the great spiritual tension without which a man called upon 'to come before the people' is unthinkable: awareness that he must communicate to the people who have come to hear him something important, significant, deep, different from the daily humdrum experiences, thoughts, and feelings. This type of nervousness is a good and necessary feeling and anyone incapable of it, who walks on to the platform as a good official walks into his office certain that today, too, he will perform the tasks required of him, such a person cannot be a true artist.[21]

Neuhaus was a great teacher and a man of deep wisdom, and I find it hard to disagree with his views. I am aware that by agreeing with both Alexander and Neuhaus I hold two opposite views on the same subject. Neuhaus always spoke of the 'law of dialectics'. This *Webster's*

Ninth New Collegiate Dictionary defines as 'the Hegelian process of change in which a concept or its realization passes over into and is preserved and fulfilled by its opposite'. Let us note that Neuhaus's career as a concert pianist was cut short by crippling stage fright. Could it be that his career might have been saved by Alexander?

Conclusions

The Conscious Mind

In his lifetime Alexander found ardent supporters in the fields of science, education, politics, and all the arts. Among his pupils there were prominent men such as George Bernard Shaw, Aldous Huxley, John Dewey, the biologists George Coghill and Sir Charles Sherrington, and many others.

The Alexander Technique belongs squarely in the mainstream of human intellectual and practical endeavour, *however much it may depart from received wisdom*. I think we could call Alexander a great rationalist. He asserted that the triumph over the powers of all disease and disabilities 'is not to be won in sleep, in trance, in submission, in paralysis, or in anaesthesia, but in a clear, open-eyed, reasoning, deliberate consciousness and apprehension of the wonderful potentialities possessed by mankind, the transcendent inheritance of a conscious mind'.[1]

We must not forget, however, that Alexander also said: 'As a matter of fact, feeling is much more use than what they call "mind" when it's right.'[2] Reason must not be confused with intellectual head-standing which excuses and justifies the unreasonable. Let us reject this mindless 'mind', but not in favour of unreliable feeling, which is no better.

For some members of the public, as well as for a number of Alexander teachers, the Technique is part of the New Age movement, and as such it entails certain behaviours which, in my opinion, run counter to rationality. This is unfortunate in many ways. It diminishes Alexander's achievements, it dilutes and distorts his principles, and it lessens the impact the Technique could make on society at large.

A teacher cannot prevent a mystical-minded pupil from believing that the Technique deals with so-called metaphysics, but this was certainly not Alexander's intention. 'It has always seemed to me', he wrote wrily, 'that the first duty of man was and is to understand and develop these potentialities which are well within the sphere of his activities here on this earth.'[3]

Restoring the Innate

When learning the Alexander Technique you develop an utterly different way of using your whole self—different, that is, from how you use your self as a *normal, badly co-ordinated adult*. I discussed the various meanings of 'normal' and 'natural' in Chapter 17, 'Aesthetic Judgements'. You may feel that Alexandrian use is unnatural, but it would be correct only to call it non-habitual, for indeed it is natural (according to the laws of Nature). '*Re-education is not a process of adding something but of restoring something*,' wrote Alexander.[4] 'When an investigation comes to be made,' he said elsewhere, 'it will be found that every single thing we are doing in the work is exactly what is being done in Nature where the conditions are right, the difference being that we are learning to do it consciously.'[5]

'Nothing extraneous can be added to the organ of song,' wrote Husler and Rodd-Marling; '. . . all the qualities needed in singing exist already within it.' Further, they wrote, 'nothing can release these qualities except the proper functioning of the organ itself'.[6] This is so in music-making and away from it. I think it was Plato who said that you can only teach someone that which he knows already. The Alexander Technique gives you something that was yours all along. Yet in rediscovering your true self you become utterly different from who you are today.

Personal Responsibility, Self-Restraint, and Control

I wrote in the Introduction about the various causes that have been advanced for our problems: stress, human design, civilization, *other people*. Alexander made a point we should all bear in mind at all times: 'If we face the facts, every honest man and woman on this earth today must admit that each and every one of us is more or less responsible for what is happening at this moment.'[7] Patrick Macdonald sees the issue in a similar light, asserting that all the causes of his misuse notwithstanding, 'a pupil should accept personal responsibility for the mess he is in. And what is more important, he should accept responsibility for getting himself out of it.'[8]

Macdonald's words are forward-looking. To accept responsibility for your own choices, decisions, and reactions and the consequences they entail is an extremely liberating act of self-affirmation. It turns a situation of dependency and weakness into one full of possibilities—for growth and change, and for control of your own life. It is not always easy to take charge, particularly in Alexander's non-doing way. Yet you have no choice but to take charge. Once you ease into it, though, you will never again wish that somebody else controlled your life for you.

We have seen that cause, effect, and remedy become, in Alexander's understanding, end-gaining, misuse, and inhibition. This last is the only way to eliminate end-gaining, and as such is the cornerstone of the Technique. 'Boiled down,' Alexander wrote, 'it all comes to inhibiting a particular reaction to a given stimulus. But no one will see it that way. They will all see it as getting in and out of a chair the right way. It is nothing of the kind. It is that a pupil decides what he will or will not consent to do.'[9]

In Chapter 4, 'Inhibition', I wrote that inhibition is a form of self-denial. You deny yourself your habitual reaction: you do not consent to pull down, and choose to think up instead. To some the combination of responsibility and self-restraint may seem a step backwards, after all the struggles we have gone through in our search for individual freedom and self-expression. Yet we cannot deny that many of our problems today, individually and collectively, result from our insistence on the instant gratification of every desire, however unnatural.

We need to redefine freedom. Since instant gratification is often automatic and addictive, you cannot consider yourself a free person until you are able to restrain yourself from it, by choice, at any time, in any situation. Thus self-restraint becomes a precondition of freedom. Besides helping you fulfil your true nature, self-restraint (as practised in the Alexander Technique) is enormous fun—more gratifying than instant gratification could ever be. 'If only so many uncontrolled things did not coexist within us,' wrote Wilhelm Furtwängler, 'then that which is controlled would no longer be worth the effort!'[10]

The issues of freedom and control are closely intertwined. I discussed Alexander's understanding of control in Chapter 2, 'The Primary

Control'. Of direct control of bodily functions, Alexander wrote that 'if such a thing were possible, and if I could endow any person with such power tomorrow, I should know perfectly well that I should, by so doing, be signing that person's death warrant'.[11] We tend to think of control as turning something on and off, like an electrical appliance. 'Control', Alexander said, 'should be in process, not superimposed.'[12] His conception of control 'does not necessarily imply any distinction between the thing controlled and the control itself'.[13] A committed study of the Technique does give you a great deal of control, but only after you give up preconceived ideas of control. Alexandrian control manifests itself not in things that you do, but in things that you stop doing—a point which you will understand after experiencing it.

Limits of the Technique

Throughout the book I have focused, naturally enough, on the framework of the Alexander Technique. This says that use affects functioning; end-gaining causes misuse of the self; and inhibition of end-gaining desires and of their attendant interference with the Primary Control is the key to solving any problems—'physical' or 'mental', technical or musical.

This framework is extremely powerful, yet we must accept that the Technique has its limitations. By this I do not mean the inadequacies ensuing from taking half a dozen Alexander lessons from an inexperienced teacher. To judge a theory objectively, you must consider an in-depth application of its principles and procedures under ideal conditions.

Even under the best conditions, however, there are things that the Technique will never accomplish. 'You can't change the course of nature by co-ordinating yourself,' said Alexander.[14] In the Introduction I spoke somewhat dismissively of 'the piecemeal approaches of psychotherapy, physiotherapy, surgery, drugs, ergonomics, and firing the conductor'. I wanted to highlight the differences between the Alexander Technique and these other ways of dealing with problems. The importance of your use notwithstanding, there will always be difficulties that can be successfully dealt with *only* through drugs, surgery, or, indeed, firing the conductor. But discussing these problems is outside the scope of this book.

The Alexander Technique can only help you become your best. It may happen, however, that your best does not make you a world-class concert artist. A committed study of the Alexander Technique will help you discover and develop your potentialities, and no more. Keep in mind, however, that you (and your family and teachers) have always assessed your talents in light of your habitual misuse. Not until you have freed your use from the constraints of habit and faulty sensory awareness will you know how far you can really go.

Theory and Practice

Alexander never set out to create a philosophy or a school of thought. What motivated him was the need to find a practical solution to a real-life problem. 'We are forced in our teaching at every point to translate theories into concrete processes,'[15] he said. Yet the practicalness of the Alexander Technique is made all the more impressive by the breadth and depth of its principles. You cannot practise the 'technique' separately from its principles. Alexander wrote:

The difficulty for all of us is to take up a new way of life in which we must apply principles instead of the haphazard end-gaining methods of the past. This indicates a slow process and we must all be content with steady improvements from day to day; but we must see to it that *we are really depending upon the application of our principles in all our endeavours in every direction from day to day.*[16]

Many of my readers may be put off by the jargon of the Technique, by the claims made for it by Alexander and others (including myself), and by the way the Technique seems to negate some cherished beliefs. Yet it would be unfair to judge the Technique by its intellectual framework (as I present it) alone. *Unless you test something, and until you master it, you do not have the right to an opinion.* To find out if you 'like' the Alexander Technique and if you 'believe' in it, you must *try it* and *master it* first. Judge it not by its theories as I state them in this book, but by the effects of a committed, practical study of it.

A Long Road

A wise man said long ago, 'The unexamined life is not worth living.' The Alexander Technique is not the only way of examining your life, but it certainly is efficient, true to Nature, all-encompassing, and great fun. I do not think you have to learn the Technique to fulfil your potential and to be healthy and happy, but I do believe that to achieve these goals you have to go through a journey of self-discovery and transformation. If it is to take you forwards and upwards from where you are today, this journey, however undertaken, will inevitably share some characteristics with Alexander's.

Alexander used to say that 'there is no royal road to anything worth having'. At the end of his long life, he was asked if he ever stopped working on himself. 'I dare not,' he replied. Anybody who says that it is easy to learn the Technique is fooling himself. A brief introductory course of lessons sometimes produces startling results, yet the force of habit, and the faulty sensory awareness inseparable from it, cannot be overestimated.

Musicians accept that theirs is a long and difficult journey. Ferruccio Busoni, considered to be the first great modern pianist, said of practising the piano that it is 'like an animal whose heads are continually growing again, however many one cuts off'.[17] Maurice Ravel attended Gabriel Fauré's composition class at the Paris Conservatoire even after he had written his magnificent String Quartet. Lotte Lehmann, at the end of her distinguished singing career, would still take forty-five minutes every day to execute a single, perfect slow scale. Nadia Boulanger, the outstanding teacher of composition and musical analysis, could be found practising simple keyboard harmony exercises in her ripe old age.

These brilliant artists, men and women of exceptional talent, worked long and hard at the basics of their skills. Can we, badly co-ordinated musicians of average ability, achieve anything in six easy lessons? I do not think so. To co-ordinate yourself, to learn and change and grow, *to pass from the known to the unknown*: there is no worthier goal and no greater adventure. There is nothing harder in life either.

Alexander the rogue liked saying, 'We can throw away the habit of a lifetime in a few minutes if we use our brains.'[18] It is entirely true. The catch is that it takes us a lifetime to learn how to use our brains.

Appendix A

The Medical Perspective

In Chapter 7, 'The Lesson', I argued that the Alexander Technique is not a therapy but an education. Yet consider this: musicians seek the Technique after having been diagnosed as suffering from conditions such as tendonitis, bursitis, lordosis, scoliosis, tennis elbow, RSI, carpal tunnel syndrome, slipped disks, hernia, lumbago, sciatica, osteoporosis, arthritis, and rheumatism. (For the sake of argument I limit myself here to a partial list of skeletal and muscular conditions. Pupils seek the Technique for many other reasons as well, including so-called 'mental problems'. Further, 'there is no real separation between mind and body,' as Norman Cousins wrote; 'illness is always an interaction between both.'[1]) They come to the Technique because they are suffering discomfort or even disabling pain. After a course of lessons in the Technique they cease to suffer pain, and they cease to be diagnosed as having tendonitis or whatever else.

Today lessons in the Technique are offered in some clinics in Great Britain's National Health Service. Some private insurers reimburse their subscribers' Alexander lessons. Doctors and other scientists have long supported the Technique. Nikolaas Tinbergen devoted part of his oration accepting the 1973 Nobel Prize for Physiology or Medicine to a discussion of the therapeutic benefits of the Technique. Is it, then, a therapy or not?

This is more than semantics. Therapy entails different aims and methods from education, and the relationship between teacher and pupil demands different attitudes, of both participants, from that between therapist and client. I believe that the Technique serves the public better, and is better served by the public, if Alexander teachers continue to think of themselves and to present themselves as teachers. A good Alexander teacher does not aim to treat or cure illness. Indeed, she veers you away from even wishing to solve a specific problem directly. Instead she leads you through a series of *indirect procedures* that address not specific ills but a state of total co-ordination or use of the self.

It is possible for somebody to suffer from backache not because of misuse, but because of cancer, for instance, or other diseases which can only be detected through extensive testing and through diagnostic tools which are outside the training of an Alexander teacher. Indeed, there are conditions for which modern medicine offers the best possible treatment.

Yet this does not invalidate the Technique in any way. Sometimes use of the self is the main or sole cause of disease. At other times it plays a secondary or indirect role. Even when use of the self plays no role in the onset of a medical problem (following a car accident, for instance), it certainly plays a role in the way a patient responds to illness and treatment. Good doctors have always known so, although they usually talk of 'attitude', 'character', or 'will' rather than use of the self. And yet modern medicine has had to 'discover' this. In Norman Cousins's modern classic, *Anatomy of an Illness as Perceived by the Patient*, the excitement and astonishment expressed at the power of the organism to regenerate itself, genuine as it may be, is but puzzling to a commonsensical observer. Of course different attitudes to illness (and to life) will entail different responses to therapy! I consider this no more than a truism; the real question has always been how to become aware of your own attitudes and how to change them when they are inadequate.

'The regenerative and restorative force in human beings is at the core of human uniqueness,' wrote Cousins. 'Sometimes this force is blocked or underdeveloped.'[2] The Alexander Technique effectively unblocks and develops this force. I hope that my book as a whole argues this point convincingly.

'Health in living', Alexander wrote, 'may be defined as the best possible reaction of the organism to the stimuli of living as manifested in its use and functioning.'[3] Diet, smoking, drinking, exercise, interpersonal relationships, upbringing, and good old genetics all play a role in health and disease. The use of the self, however, is a constant in everything you do. Exercise, for instance, is beneficial only to the extent that you use yourself well when exercising. Changing your use sometimes entails automatic, *indirect* changes to your habits of eating and drinking. Awareness of your use should also permeate intentional, *direct* efforts at altering your lifestyle; it is your good use that will make any changes operative and long-lasting. And the way you use yourself—what Alexander called your 'individuality and character'—definitely determines the way you react to others, and others to you. Use yourself well, in everything that you do, and you will be healthy indeed.

I have spoken of the use of the self in the onset of illness and in therapy. Ideally, good use prevents illness. Medical science today gives us much knowledge about the prevention of disease. The Alexander Technique enlarges this knowledge, and allows us to put it into practice.

In summary, the Technique is an education that has therapeutic effects. 'Education in the widest sense of the word', wrote Alexander, ' . . . deals with the control of human reaction.'[4] Personal responsibility for your own reactions (and therefore for your own well-being) is the ultimate goal of education, and preventing things from ever going wrong the ultimate goal of personal responsibility.

Appendix B

Questions and Answers

How do I find a teacher?

The Society of Teachers of the Alexander Technique was founded in London in 1958. It congregates professionally trained teachers world-wide, and it will send you a list of qualified teachers upon request. Several countries have national teachers' associations that are affiliated to STAT; STAT's list includes their addresses. Here I limit myself to the addresses of the American and Canadian societies, as well as STAT. There exist teachers and training courses that are not affiliated to STAT.

STAT
20 London House
266 Fulham Road
London SW10 9EL
United Kingdom
Telephone: (0171) 351 0828; fax: (0171) 352 1556

NASTAT
PO Box 517
Urbana IL 61801-0517
USA
Telephone: (800) 473 0620; (310) 827 8106

CANSTAT
Box 47025, Apt. 12
555 West 12th Avenue
Vancouver, B. C. V5Z 3XO
CANADA
Telephone: (604) 689 9102

How will I know if my teacher is good?

The Alexander Technique, like all other professions in the world, is peopled by men and women of widely varying ability. One would not assume that all members of the American Medical Association, for instance, are equally good doctors.

In truth it is quite difficult to assess Alexander teachers. Experience and seniority are not necessarily indicative of insight or ability. A pleasant manner is not always the sign of a competent professional; a good pedagogue may happen to have a difficult temperament.

In an unpublished paper, Patrick Macdonald wrote of the requirements of good teaching. Among other qualities, he argued, a teacher should have the 'ability to explain to pupils what they should not do, what they should do and how they should do it, and how they should continue to do it in the absence of a teacher'. Macdonald added that 'the teacher must know what the pupil is doing, what he himself is doing, what he is going to try and do and how he is going to do it. He should also see to it to the best of his ability that he (the teacher) is doing what he thinks he is doing and not something quite different.' Finally, he quoted Irene Tasker, one of Alexander's first assistants: 'The criterion of good teaching is whether you have changed your pupil's thinking.'[1]

These guidelines are thoroughly sensible, yet you will need a certain amount of Alexander experience before you can tell what your teacher is trying to do, and whether or not she is succeeding. In effect, there are no easy ways of assessing your teacher's competence. If you can not rely on a recommendation from somebody you know, use your common sense, discernment, and intuition, but do not forget that, thanks to faulty sensory awareness, you may be wrong. Keep in mind, too, that just as you change music teachers from time to time, you can and should change Alexander teachers as need dictates it.

There are no teachers in my town. What should I do?

Get together a group of like-minded friends and colleagues and invite an Alexander teacher to come to your town for a series of lectures, lessons, and workshops. Most national associations (like STAT and NASTAT) publish regular newsletters where you can advertise for a visiting teacher.

I have long tried to invite an Alexander teacher to my town, to no avail. What can I do?

In some circumstances it may be truly impossible to get hold of an Alexander teacher. Here I remind you of one of my conclusions: the Alexander Technique is a great way forwards and upwards, but not the only one. The Technique is a manifestation of a certain outlook in life. If you cannot find an Alexander teacher, look for someone else whose outlook is in harmony with Alexander's. I have had teachers of aikido and of singing, for instance, whose work was suffused with the principles of the Technique, even though these teachers had never done any Alexander work. The Technique is based upon universal principles that inevitably crop up in other spheres of knowledge and activity. I need not describe all these principles here. Work from the general to the particular; attempt not do the right thing, but to stop doing the wrong thing; seek not relaxation, but necessary tension. Keep in mind that ends condition means indirectly, but means condition ends directly. You must therefore always stick to the right means.

It could be that, in the absence of an Alexander teacher, a master potter, a dancer, a martial artist, an enlightened priest would help you along the right path. But—how to find them? I wish I knew.

How many lessons will I need?

It has been said that you can learn the basics of the Alexander Technique in some twenty-five lessons. Personally I do not believe it is possible to state a specific number of lessons as 'right' or 'needed' or 'enough' for any one pupil. Once I told a beginner that at the end of a year of lessons he would have a good idea of what the Technique could do for him. Vague as it may be, this is honest and realistic. Remember Alexander's words: there is no royal road to anything worth having.

You could learn to play 'Chopsticks' at the piano in thirty seconds. It would take you rather longer to become a concert pianist. Learning the Alexander Technique is no different. There is no limit to how far you can take the Technique in your life. The number of lessons you will need will depend on your needs and desires, your general health, your open-mindedness, your capacity for laughing at yourself when you go wrong, and much else besides.

Is the Technique ever harmful?

If you find yourself in the hands of an incompetent professional—be he a doctor, mechanic, stockbroker, or Alexander teacher—then you are in for some trouble. This is not the same as saying that the Technique is actually harmful, for in itself it never is.

People who ask the question above often really mean to ask, 'What are the risks associated with the Technique?' Throughout I have written about some of the difficulties involved in learning the Technique, and how better to overcome them. Here I wish to consider a single aspect of the Technique.

Perhaps you have always been unaware of your misuse. To feel, suddenly and accurately, all that is wrong in what you do and not being able to fix it may be very upsetting. Before arriving at self-awareness, you need to pass through self-consciousness. If you do not persevere, you risk *staying* self-conscious and regretting the loss of your innocence.

To study the Alexander Technique is to pass from the known to the unknown, the known being wrong and the unknown, right. The passage is available to all, but for some the journey entails greater sacrifice than for others. It may appear to them that they are being asked to make a choice between doing what is right and being happy. In truth the choice is between relative happiness today and greater happiness later, after a time of possible unhappiness.

I would not give up the Technique for anything in this world. Yet I have come to believe, as a teacher, that some people are better off staying as they are today. Where ignorance is bliss, 'tis folly to be wise.

Are there people who do not need the Technique?

There is no situation in which the Technique ceases being applicable. People who are naturally and wholly healthy, enlightened, and happy, could use the Technique to strengthen their well-being, to prevent the onset of disease, to widen their horizons, to help others, or simply to have a good time.

Such people, however, are extremely rare. A case more to the point would be a musician who, despite misusing himself, is healthy and successful, and therefore not in apparent need of the Alexander Technique. Several possibilities exist:

1. He is well today, but his misuse will one day catch up with him and start to give him trouble.

2. He is well, but could be better still. 'Normal health' is not 'ideal health'. True freedom and well-being are hard to imagine for people who are contented with being moderately healthy.

3. He is well, but at a price: taking medicine regularly, perhaps. The population of France is considered among the healthiest today. Yet an average of 38 prescriptions are dispensed per inhabitant, per year—the highest consumption of drugs in the world. I see a little contradiction here.

4. The musician of our example plays well and is professionally successful. This does not mean that he could not play better still, or be yet more successful.

5. He plays well enough today, but his playing, and his career, may deteriorate at some point. Indeed, this has happened to many fine musicians, who start promising careers but who eventually 'lose their touch'. Talent and will-power are not enough, particularly when youth—source of great miracles—runs out.

6. He plays well, but teaches badly. Again, this is the case with many musicians, prominent pedagogues included.

In each of these hypothetical situations the Alexander Technique would play a positive role: to allow someone who is well to stay well or become better still, to allow a performer to become a better teacher, and so on.

My Alexander teacher disagrees with every word in this book.
How can that be?

Patrick Macdonald, my beloved teacher, entitled his book *The Alexander Technique as I See it*. Most books written about most subjects should include this little 'as I see it' in their title. There is no unanimity on anything in this world— and a good thing it is, too.

Appendix C

F. M. Alexander: A Biographical Sketch

Frederick Matthias Alexander, called F. M. by all who knew him, was born at Wynyard, on the north-west coast of Tasmania, in 1869. He spent part of his childhood on his grandfather's country estate, where he developed his lifelong love of horses.

At the age of 20 Alexander moved to Melbourne, where he pursued a career as an actor specializing in reciting. He was successful early on, and toured Australia and Tasmania. Nevertheless, he was hampered by vocal problems, in particular hoarseness on stage. Doctors and vocal experts were unable to help him. Faced with the prospect of unreliable and possibly harmful surgery, Alexander, in a stroke of genius, decided instead to find out what he was doing to himself that was causing his troubles. His search led him to the discoveries that gave rise to the teaching technique that now bears his name. The first chapter of his book *The Use of the Self* is given over to a full account of his research, and is required reading for all Alexandrians.

His various travels in Australia and New Zealand culminated in a move to Sydney, where his teaching practice flourished. He directed the Sydney Dramatic and Operatic Conservatorium between 1900 and 1904, when he moved to England.

A story is told of Alexander putting his last £5 on a 150–1 bet at the horse races. The subsequent win was instrumental in helping his settling in London. Betting on horses remained one of his passions, in which he indulged intemperately.

In the years before World War I, Alexander worked mainly with actors, including many prominent ones. Indeed, throughout his life Alexander met with great success as a teacher, and counted among his pupils George Bernard Shaw, Aldous Huxley, Sir Stafford Cripps (Chancellor of the Exchequer in the 1940s), and other luminaries.

He published his first book, *Man's Supreme Inheritance*, in 1910. From 1914 to 1924 he shared his time between England and the USA and wrote two further books, *Conscious Control* and *Constructive Conscious Control of the Individual*. Later they were amalgamated and republished under the second title. During this time Alexander started his friendship with John Dewey, the American philosopher, who was strongly influenced by Alexander's teachings.

Alexander ran a teacher-training course from 1930 to 1940, when he moved to America on account of the war. His third book, *The Use of the Self*, came out in 1932, and his fourth and last, *The Universal Constant in Living*, in 1941.

Alexander returned to England in 1943, and resumed training teachers in 1945.

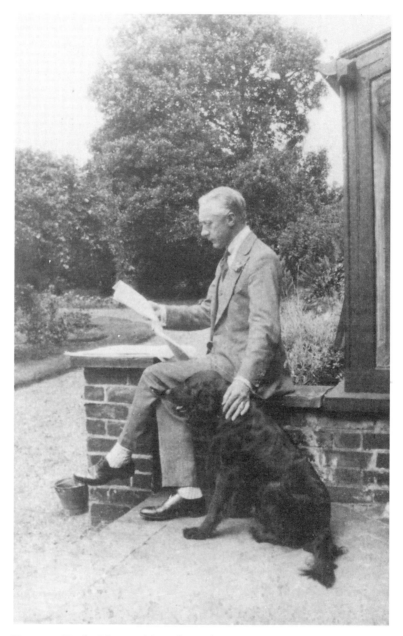

FIG. 23. Frederick Matthias Alexander (1869–1955)

In 1948, after his work was attacked in an official publication, he brought a libel action against the South African government. He won damages and costs, but the drawn-out trial caused him much suffering. He died in 1955, aged 86 and in full possession of his faculties, having worked until a few days before his death.

Alexander's four books are kept intermittently in print, in various British and American editions. They are not easy to grasp, particularly for us modern readers with short attention spans. Committed Alexandrians should make a serious study of these texts, not because they come from the pen of an infallible sage, but because they are full of well-argued insights and instructive anecdotes. Reading the books and taking lessons from a qualified teacher should be complementary experiences.

Alexander was one of the century's great freethinkers, and his discoveries should be dearly cherished by all. Yet he was also a somewhat injudicious man who, in Dr Wilfred Barlow's words, 'tended to get himself involved in a complicated network of financial and social transactions'.[1] Some teachers who knew him—notably Lulie Westfeld, Walter Carrington, and Frank Pierce Jones—have also written of the shortcomings of Alexander the pedagogue and spokesman.

Alexander's idiosyncrasies notwithstanding, his discoveries are of universal importance. Society at large has yet to give Alexander his due; end-gaining and faulty sensory awareness lead us to deny our self-inflicted problems and ignore the solutions that he proposed. I pay joyful homage to a great man, and hope that my readers too will have reasons to thank Alexander for a marvellous legacy.

Appendix D
My Pantheon

Throughout this book I have mentioned many musicians as I have argued various points about the Alexander Technique. Sometimes I have quoted them (Furtwängler, Neuhaus, Boulanger, and so on). At times I have quoted from their biographies (Busoni, for instance). On occasion I have showed their pictures (Rubinstein, Casals, Stokowski, and others). A few times I have referred the reader to records and videos of their performances (Primrose, Rubinstein, Busoni). Yet the reader may fail to appreciate my arguments about the Alexander Technique if he remains unfamiliar with the musicians I hold as exemplars.

A detailed discussion of their lives and the historical forces that acted upon them and were shaped by them in turn would be outside the scope of this book. Instead I wish to say a few words about some of these musicians. Quite capriciously, I have chosen to limit myself to seven of them. (Did you ever hear of a film called *The Six Samurai*? I didn't think so.) To be comprehensive would be both difficult and unnecessary: my vignettes, brief and incomplete, are meant to stimulate your curiosity and encourage you to undertake your own, neverending research. I hope you will go on to read about these and other musicians and collect their recordings and videos.

Nadia Boulanger (b. Paris, 1887; d. Paris, 1979) was a pianist, composer, conductor, and pedagogue. She pioneered the modern rediscovery of Claudio Monteverdi, recording a series of madrigals with her vocal ensemble in 1937. She was the first woman to conduct a complete performance of the Royal Philharmonic Society in London, also in 1937. Boulanger's signal achievement was as a teacher of composition and music theory. Her pupils include Aaron Copland, Walter Piston, Eliot Carter, Lennox Berkeley, and dozens of other accomplished instrumentalists, singers, composers, and conductors. Boulanger has also left a recorded legacy as pianist and conductor. You may wish to hear her 1948 recording of Gabriel Fauré's Requiem as well as a selection of Monteverdi madrigals, reissued on CD.[1] Listen too to the delightful waltzes by Johannes Brahms which Boulanger recorded with Dinu Lipatti, one of her great pupils and a pianist with whom you should also become familiar. These waltzes are included in a CD of Lipatti's performances,[2] together with works by Chopin, Liszt, Ravel, and Enescu.

Ferruccio Busoni (b. Empoli, Italy, 1866; d. Berlin, 1924) is considered by many to have been the first great modern pianist, whose virtuosity and brilliance may have been equalled but not surpassed. Nadia Boulanger described a few aspects of his playing: '[His] articulation was perfect, and came not only from the astonishing evenness of his technique, but above all from his prodigious sense of rhythm. . . . He played in a singular way, with the air of composing as he played.'[3] To my mind this describes an ideal performer, whom we all would do well to emulate. Busoni was a noted pedagogue and prolific composer, whose visionary works are only now becoming widely appreciated. In Chapter 10, 'The Arms and Hands', I have given the details of his sole surviving recording.

Pablo Casals (b. Vendrell, Catalonia, 1876; d. Rio Piedras, Puerto Rico, 1973) was a pianist, composer, and conductor, but his greatest contribution to the history of music was as a cellist. He revolutionized cello technique and sound-production, re-established Bach's Suites for unaccompanied cello as staples of the repertoire, and taught several fine cellists. He left many recordings as recitalist, concerto soloist, chamber musician, conductor, and composer. There exist also videos of his master-classes, in which his use at the cello is a joy to behold.

Wilhelm Furtwängler (b. Berlin, 1886; d. near Baden-Baden, 1954) conducted many of the great orchestras all over the world, but his longest tenures were at the Berlin Philharmonic, from 1922 to the end of his life, and at the Vienna Philharmonic, in 1927–30 and 1947–54. He remained in Germany during World War II, and the end of his life was dogged by political controversy. Although he was cleared of pro-Nazi activities in 1946, American activists kept him out of the USA after the war. You may wish to engage in an old game that musicians play among themselves, which consists of comparing Furtwängler with Arturo Toscanini (b. Parma, 1867; d. New York, 1957) and siding passionately with one against the other. Furtwängler's recordings and his writings both deserve scrutiny. A superb filmed documentary, *The Art of Conducting: Great Conductors of the Past*, available on the Teldec label (distributed by BMG), includes a few minutes of his artistry. I shall return to this documentary shortly.

Heinrich Neuhaus (b. Elisavetgrad, Ukraine, 1888; d. Moscow, 1964) had a distinguished career as a pianist, but, like Boulanger, will be remembered first and foremost as a great teacher. His students include Sviatoslav Richter, Emil Gilels, and Radu Lupu, to cite only those that became well-known in the West. There exists a CD of Neuhaus performing works by Mozart, Debussy, and Prokofiev.[4]

The playing of Artur Rubinstein (b. Łódź, Poland, 1887; d. Geneva, 1982), more than anyone else's, seemed to embody to perfection all the principles of the Alexander Technique and the artistic outlook these principles entail. A child prodigy whose education was at one point supervised by Joseph Joachim (who premièred Brahms's Concerto for violin and orchestra), Rubinstein went on to a brilliant, all-encompassing career as recitalist, soloist, and chamber musician. He was a terrific raconteur, and his volumes of autobiography tell amusingly of a life which we mere mortals can barely imagine. There exist many recordings and videos of Rubinstein. Besides the recital mentioned in Chapter 10, 'The Arms and Hands', you may wish to study his performance of concertos by Grieg, Chopin, and Saint-Saëns, available in a Decca/Polygram video.

Leopold Stokowski (b. London, 1882; d. Nether Wallop, Hants., 1977) had a long and distinguished career, the cornerstone of which was his stewardship of the Philadelphia Symphony Orchestra from 1912 to 1938. Every conductor obtains a particular sound from the orchestras they work with; this is but a truism. Yet Stokowski's sound was more remarkable and individual than most; indeed, some critics question both his unique orchestral voice and the very means whereby he obtained it, maintaining that he took undue liberties with the musical text. Stokowski was a champion of modern music, a keen student of recording techniques, and a master showman. He conducted the music for Walt Disney's *Fantasia*, and, again, some critics think the less of him for it. (I think the less of those critics for that.) He too can be found on the documentary *The Art of Conducting: Great Conductors of the Past*. I have never seen somebody use himself better, with greater economy, elegance, or intelligence. The resulting orchestral sound and rhythmic forward motion speak for themselves.

You may have noticed that the majority of the musicians above died in their eighties and nineties. This makes sense in light of the Alexander Technique. (Alexander himself was 86 when he died.) If indeed these men and women embody healthy principles of use and attitude, then it is logical that they should live long, productive lives.

You may also have wondered whether I only admire dead people. Not at all; simply for the purposes of this discussion, I have limited myself to figures whose lives we can consider with a little distance. Some of my other beloved models are only two or three years old.

Finally, you may argue, after listening to the records I mention, that you do not actually like them. We need not agree on our likes and dislikes, but to have a meaningful discussion about artistic outlook and taste we both need to be well informed. To inform, not to convince, is the sole purpose of this appendix. (I have tried to convince you elsewhere in the book.)

Notes

Introduction

1. *Anatomy of an Illness as Perceived by the Patient: Reflections on Healing and Regeneration* (New York: Bantam Books, 1981), 65.
2. David Dalton, *Playing the Viola: Conversations with William Primrose* (Oxford: Oxford University Press, 1988), 7.
3. Trans. K. A. Leibovitch (London: Barrie and Jenkins, 1973), 72.
4. Ibid. 109–11 (my italics).
5. II. ii.
6. *MSI* 91.
7. Richard Williams, 'Age of the Rocket Man', *Independent on Sunday Review* (20 June 1993), 11.

Chapter 1

1. Wilhelm Furtwängler, *Notebooks 1924–1954*, trans. Shaun Whiteside, ed. and with an Introduction by Michael Tanner (London: Quartet Books, 1989), 73.
2. *The Man who Mistook his Wife for a Hat and Other Clinical Tales* (New York: Harper Perennial, 1990), 93.
3. *The Integrative Action of the Nervous System*, 2nd edn. (New Haven: Yale University Press, 1961), p. xvi.
4. Ibid. 14.
5. *MSI* 23.
6. *US* 2.
7. *RB* 2.
8. In Steve Conner, 'The Brain Machines', *Independent on Sunday Review* (7 Nov. 1993), 76.
9. *The Art of Piano Playing*, 87.
10. 'Appreciation', in Alexander, *UCL*, p. xxi.
11. *RB* 4.
12. *The Art of Piano Playing*, 101.
13. Ibid. 105.
14. *Vocal Wisdom: Maxims Transcribed and Edited by William Earl Brown* (New York: Taplinger Publishing Co. Inc., 1931), 29.
15. Ibid. 63.
16. *The Alexander Technique as I See it* (Brighton: Rahula Books, 1989), 30.

17. *The Free Voice: A Guide to Natural Singing* (New York: Joseph Patelson Music House, 1972), 12.
18. *Singing: The Physical Nature of the Vocal Organ. A Guide to the Unlocking of the Singing Voice* (London: Faber and Faber Ltd., 1965), 72.
19. *Ride with your Mind: A Right Brain Approach to Riding* (London: The Kingswood Press, 1991), p. xvi.
20. *UCL* 106.
21. *Body Awareness in Action: A Study of the Alexander Technique*, with an Introduction by J. McVicker Hunt (New York: Schocken Books, 1976), 195.
22. *UCL*, p. xl.
23. Ibid. 10.
24. By Peter Wingate, with Richard Wingate, 3rd edn. (London: Penguin Books, 1988), 96.

Chapter 2

1. 'Appreciation', p. xxviii.
2. Margaret E. Hogg, *A Biology of Man*, vol. ii: *Man the Animal* (London: Heinemann Educational Books, 1966), 41.
3. Ibid. 50.
4. Ibid. 54.
5. *USE* 28.
6. Ibid. 27.
7. *UCL* 185.
8. *RB* 3.
9. *CCC* 10 n.
10. *Essays on the Nature of Singing* (Huntsville, Tex.: Recital Publications, 1992), 59.
11. *Cello Technique: Principles and Forms of Movement*, trans. Barbara Haimberger Thiem (Bloomington, Ind.: Indiana University Press, 1975), 3.
12. (London: Rockliff, 1958), 1.
13. *MSI* 120.

Chapter 3

1. *RB* 10.
2. Ibid. 6.
3. *CCC* 146.
4. *The Free Voice*, 86.
5. *The Man who Mistook*, 49.
6. Ibid. 74.
7. Ibid. 72.
8. Ibid.

9. 'Appreciation', p. xxiii.
10. Quoted by Sacks, *The Man who Mistook*, 73.
11. *UCL* 110.

Chapter 4

1. *UCL* 7.
2. Quoted ibid. 110.
3. *Singing*, 5.
4. Quoted by Alexander, *UCL* 110.
5. *La dinamica del violinista* (Buenos Aires: Ricordi Americana, 1947), 36 (my trans.).
6. *The Alexander Technique*, 25.
7. Ibid. 36.
8. Ibid. 27.
9. *RB* 3.
10. *MSI* 21.

Chapter 5

1. *The Alexander Technique*, 78
2. *US* 39.
3. Ibid. 13.
4. *Cello Technique*, 3.
5. *An Epitome of the Laws of Pianoforte Technique, being a Summary Abstracted from 'The Visible and Invisible', a Digest of the Author's Technical Writings* (London: Humphrey Milford, 1931; repr. London: Oxford University Press, 1972), p. viii.
6. *The Alexander Technique*, 5.
7. Ibid. 65.
8. *Vocal Wisdom*, 29.
9. Ibid. 63.
10. *CCC* 157.
11. *MSI* 122.
12. *The Alexander Technique*, 14.
13. *RB* 8.
14. Ibid. 9.
15. *The Alexander Technique*, 2.
16. *The Tao of Jeet Kune Do* (Burbank, Calif.: Ohara Publications, Inc., 1975), 21.
17. Ibid. 203.
18. Helena Matheopoulos, *Maestro: Encounters with Conductors of Today* (London: Hutchinson, 1982), 446.

19. Review of Jonathan Drake, *Body Know-how*, Drake, *Alexander Journal*, 12 (autumn 1992), 48.

Chapter 6

1. *CCC* 209.
2. *The Alexander Technique*, 1.
3. *UCL* 105.
4. *US* 37–8.
5. *CCC* 215 (my italics).
6. *RB* 9.
7. *The Tao*, 8.
8. Ibid. 12.
9. *My Life*, with Ida Cook (London: Macdonald and Jane's, 1979), 72.
10. Hiroide Ogawa, *Enlightenment through the Art of Basketball*, trans. H. Taniguchi, James N. Delavaye, and Otis McCrail, with images by Peter Nuttall (Cambridge and New York: The Oleander Press, 1979), pages not numbered.
11. *Singing*, 107.
12. *The Free Voice*, 97.
13. *The Tao*, 12.

Chapter 7

1. *On the Alexander Technique, in Discussion with Séan Carey* (London: Sheildrake Press, 1986), 52.
2. Quoted by Alexander, *UCL* 110.
3. *RB* 4.
4. Ibid. 9.
5. *The Alexander Technique*, 13.
6. Ibid. 34.
7. *The Free Voice*, 129.
8. *CCC* 149.

Chapter 8

1. Vernon E. Krahl, 'Anatomy of the Mammalian lung', in Wallace O. Fenn and Hermann Rahn, eds., *Handbook of Physiology: A Critical, Comprehensive Presentation of Physiological Knowledge and Concepts*, iii: *Respiration* (Washington, DC: American Physiological Society, 1964), 213.
2. Emilio Agostini, 'Action of the Respiratory Muscles', ibid. 381.
3. Jere Mead and Emilio Agostini, 'Dynamics of Breathing', ibid. 421.

4. *A Dictionary of Vocal Terminology: An Analysis* (New York: Joseph Patelson Music House, 1983), 88.
5. *RB* 11.
6. *MSI* 33.
7. *Singing*, 47.
8. Wingate and Wingate, 406.
9. *A Dictionary of Vocal Terminology*, 42.
10. Ibid.
11. *CCC* 200 (my italics).
12. *A Dictionary of Vocal Terminology*, 42.
13. *Singing*, 42.
14. *Vocal Wisdom*, 134.
15. *A Dictionary of Vocal Terminology*, 42.
16. *The Voice Book* (London: Faber and Faber, 1989), 39.
17. Ibid. 37.
18. *English, French, German, and Italian Techniques of Singing: A Study in National Tonal Preferences and how they Relate to Functional Efficiency* (Metuchen, NJ: The Scarecrow Press, 1977), 40.
19. *Essays on the Nature of Singing*, 190.
20. *CCC* 193.
21. *MSI* 188.
22. *Essays on the Nature of Singing*, 168.
23. *MSI* 202.
24. Ibid. 195.
25. Ibid. 139.
26. Ibid. 195.
27. *CCC* 201.
28. *Notebooks*, quoted in John F. Perkins, Jr., 'Historical Development of Respiratory Physiology,' in Fenn and Rahn, *Handbook of Physiology*, iii. 7.
29. *Opera medica* (Geneva: de Tournes, 1681); quoted ibid. 17.
30. *MSI* 198.
31. *Singing*, 36.
32. R. A. Cluff, 'Chronic Hyperventilation and its Treatment by Physiotherapy: Discussion Paper', *Journal of the Royal Society of Medicine*, 77 (Oct. 1984), 855, 856.
33. L. C. Lum, 'Hyperventilation and Anxiety State', *Journal of the Royal Society of Medicine*, 74 (Jan. 1981), 2.
34. *The Alexander Technique*, 6.
35. *"Deep Breathing" and Physical Culture Exercises*, in *AL* 76.
36. C. L. Reid, *Essays on the Nature of Singing*, 176.
37. *RB* 6.
38. Delbert A. Dale, *Trumpet Technique* (Oxford: Oxford University Press, 1965), 33.
39. *RB* 12.

Chapter 9

1. *RB* 6.
2. Dalton, *Playing the Viola*, 174.
3. *A Treatise on the Flute*, 2nd edn. (London: Musica Rara, 1928; repr. 1967), 420.
4. *Body Awareness in Action*, 195.
5. *The Alexander Technique*, 33.
6. Quoted in Rockstro, *A Treatise on the Flute*, 427.
7. Nancy Toff, *The Flute Book* (London: David & Charles, 1985), 81.
8. *The Alexander Technique*, 36.

Chapter 10

1. Ivan Galamian, *Principles of Violin Playing and Teaching*, 2nd edn. (Englewood Cliffs, NJ: Prentice-Hall, 1985), 5.
2. *RB* 11.
3. *The Alexander Technique*, 81.
4. *RB* 9.
5. *Cello* (Yehudi Menuhin Music Guides; London and Sydney: Macdonald & Co., 1982), 161.
6. *Oboe* (Yehudi Menuhin Music Guides; London and Sydney: Macdonald & Co., 1977), 59.
7. Works by Beethoven, Schumann, Debussy, Chopin, and Mendelssohn, recorded 15 Jan. 1975 at Ambassador College, Pasadena, Calif.; distributed by BMG.
8. Personal communication to the author.
9. *MSI* 111.
10. *Cello Technique*, 144.
11. 'An Organized Method of String Playing', in Murray Grodner, ed., *Concepts in String Playing: Reflections by Artist-Teachers at the Indiana School of Music* (Bloomington, Ind., and London: Indiana University Press, 1979), 138–9.
12. *Ferruccio Busoni: Chronicle of a European*, trans. Sandra Morris (London: Calder & Boyars, 1970), 79.
13. Works by Bach, Bach–Busoni, Beethoven–Busoni, Chopin, and Liszt, recorded 1919; Pearl GEMM CD9347.
14. *Men's Health* (July–Aug. 1995), 15.
15. Joseph Horowitz, *Conversations with Arrau* (New York: Knopf, 1982), 105.
16. *Body Awareness in Action*, 65. *Webster's Ninth New Collegiate Dictionary* defines 'ischemia' as 'localized tissue anaemia due to obstruction of arterial blood'.
17. *The Art of Piano Playing*, 72.
18. *RB* 12.

Chapter 11

1. 'Training with F. M.', *Alexander Journal*, 12 (autumn 1992), 28.
2. Goossens and Roxburgh, *Oboe*, 76.
3. Denis Wick, *Trombone Technique*, rev. edn. (London: Oxford University Press, 1973), 20.
4. Toff, *The Flute Book*, 93.
5. *Running with Style* (Mt. View, Calif.: World Publications, 1975), 36.

Chapter 12

1. *Body Awareness in Action*, 68.

Chapter 14

1. *Singing*, 125.
2. *The Art of Singing and Voice Technique: A Handbook for Voice Teachers, for Professional and Amateur Singers* (London: Calder & Boyars, 1973), 22.
3. *UCL* 105.
4. *RB* 9.
5. Horowitz, *Conversations with Arrau*, 109.

Chapter 15

1. *The Integrative Action*, p. xvi.
2. Stuckenschmidt, *Ferruccio Busoni*, 79.
3. *Principles*, 5.
4. Ibid. 2.
5. *Notebooks 1924–1954*, 9.
6. *The Art of Piano Playing*, 79.
7. *The Alexander Technique*, 23.
8. *The Art of Piano Playing*, 2.
9. Ibid. 82.
10. *Notebooks 1924–1954*, 30.
11. *Singing*, 112.
12. Matheopoulos, *Maestro*, 470.
13. *The Art of Piano Playing*, 33.
14. Joan Chissell, *Schumann*, 3rd rev. edn. (London: J. M. Dent and Sons Ltd., 1977), 23.
15. Ibid.
16. *The Art of Piano Playing*, 12.
17. Ibid. 1.

Chapter 16

1. *The Tao*, 20.
2. *UCL* 216.
3. *The Free Voice*, 135.
4. *UCL* 193.
5. *RB* 11.
6. *MSI* 44.
7. *UCL* 55.
8. *RB* 8.
9. *The Alexander Technique*, 1.
10. Quoted by Neuhaus, *The Art of Piano Playing*, 33.
11. Ibid. 32.
12. *Singing*, 107.
13. Ibid. 13.
14. *US* 34.
15. *The Alexander Technique*, 1.
16. *The Accompanist . . . and Friends: An Autobiography of André Benoist* (Neptune City, NJ: Paganiniana Publications, 1978), 284.
17. *Enlightenment*, pages not numbered.
18. *RB* 5.
19. *Notebooks 1924–1954*, 32–3.
20. *MSI* 136.
21. *The Great Pianists* (London: Victor Gollancz, 1974), 280.
22. Ibid. 283.
23. Herbert R. Axelrod, ed., *Heifetz* (Neptune City, NJ: Paganiniana Publications, 1976), 123–6.
24. *Cello*, 10.
25. *UCL* 66.
26. *The Tao*, 29.
27. *CCC* 191.
28. Ibid.
29. *MSI* 143.
30. *La dinamica del violinista*, 56.
31. *CCC* 278.
32. Ibid. 274.
33. *UCL* 114.

Chapter 17

1. *UCL* 121.
2. *Vocal Wisdom*, 139.

3. *US* 74.

4. *Running with Style*, 4.

5. *US* 56.

6. *Notebooks 1924–1954*, 139.

7. p. xxi.

8. Trans. in Nancy Wilson Ross, ed., *The World of Zen* (New York: Vintage Paperbacks, 1960), 299.

9. Horowitz, *Conversations with Arrau*, 49.

10. *MSI* 136.

11. 2nd edn., rev. Ernest Gowers (Oxford: Clarendon Press, 1965, repr. 1968), 295.

12. *Notebooks 1924–1954*, 146.

13. Ibid. 127.

14. *The Alexander Technique*, 12.

15. *The Free Voice*, 86.

16. Ibid. 18.

17. *Principles*, 4.

18. *The Free Voice*, 18.

19. Ibid. 109.

20. Ibid. 86.

21. *Notebooks 1924–1954*, 139.

22. Bruno Monsaingeon, *Mademoiselle: Conversations with Nadia Boulanger*, trans. Robyn Marsack (Manchester: Carcanet Press, 1985), 95.

23. *The Tao*, 7.

24. Monsaingeon, *Mademoiselle*, 95.

25. *The Free Voice*, 149.

26. *The Art of Piano Playing*, 73.

27. *On Piano Playing: Motion, Sound and Expression* (New York: Schirmer Books, 1981), 229.

Chapter 18

1. *US* 38 (my italics).

2. Pearl GEMM CD 9453, 1990; material first recorded 1934–9.

3. *The Art of Piano Playing*, 125.

4. *La dinamica del violinista*, 96.

5. *UCL* 216.

6. *The Tao*, 44.

7. *Practising the Piano* (London: Rockliff, 1958), 55.

8. Julie Lyonn Lieberman, *You are your Instrument* (New York: Huiski Music, 1991), 34.

9. *A Dictionary of Vocal Terminology*, 56.

10. *Oboe*, 85.

11. *The Flute Book*, 93.
12. *The Art of Piano Playing*, 88.
13. Ibid. 91.

Chapter 21

1. *Trombone Technique*, 46.
2. Ibid. 42.
3. *CCC* 209.
4. *US* 34.
5. *UCL* 105.
6. *US* 37–8.
7. *CCC* 209.
8. *Essay on the Craft of Cello-Playing*, vol. ii: *The Left Hand* (Cambridge: Cambridge University Press, 1982), 6.
9. *The Art of Singing*, 83.

Chapter 22

1. *Notebooks 1924–1954*, 121.
2. *Singing*, 4.
3. *MSI* 90.

Chapter 23

1. *RB* 9.
2. *The Art of Piano Playing*, 208.
3. *CCC* 212.
4. *UCL* 211.
5. *CCC* 210.
6. *MSI* 83.
7. Quoted by Sherrington, *The Integrative Action*, 259.
8. Sandra Blakelee, 'The Physical Roots of Emotion', *International Herald Tribune* (8 Dec. 1994), 8.
9. *MSI* 23.
10. *My Life*, 100.
11. *The Tao*, 69.
12. *UCL* 184.
13. *CCC* 222.
14. *On Piano Playing*, 220.
15. *The Tao*, 21.
16. Ibid. 203.
17. *The Art of Piano Playing*, 211.

18. *Notebooks 1924–1954*, 136.
19. Ibid. 131.
20. Wingate and Wingate, *The Penguin Medical Encyclopedia*, 64.
21. *The Art of Piano Playing*, 211.

Conclusions

1. *MSI* 142.
2. *RB* 12.
3. *CCC*, preface, pages not numbered.
4. *UCL* 190.
5. *RB* 7.
6. *Singing*, 3.
7. Quoted ibid. 237.
8. *The Alexander Technique*, 17.
9. *RB* 9.
10. *Notebooks 1924–1954*, 186.
11. *MSI* 174.
12. *RB* 3.
13. *MSI* 23.
14. *RB* 3.
15. Ibid. 7.
16. Ibid. 8 (my italics).
17. Stuckenschmidt, *Ferruccio Busoni*, 86.
18. *RB* 6.

Appendix A

1. *Anatomy of an Illness*, 56.
2. Ibid. 145.
3. *UCL* 84.
4. Ibid. 36.

Appendix B

1. Patrick Macdonald, 'Six Essentials for a Teacher of the F. Matthias Alexander Technique' (10 July 1970).

Appendix C

1. Wilfred Barlow, *The Alexander Principle*, 2nd edn. (London: Victor Gollancz, 1990), 237.

Appendix D

1. EMI CDH 7 61025 2.
2. EMI CDH 7 63038 2.
3. Monsaingeon, *Mademoiselle*, 99.
4. Melodyia 74321 25174.

Bibliography

For Frederick Matthias Alexander's writings, see Abbreviations, fo. xiii.

AXELROD, HERBERT R., ed., *Heifetz* (Neptune City, NJ: Paganiniana Publications, 1976).

BARLOW, WILFRED, *The Alexander Principle*, 2nd edn. (London: Victor Gollancz, 1990).

BENOIST, ANDRÉ, *The Accompanist . . . and Friends: An Autobiography of André Benoist* (Nepture City, NJ: Paganiniana Publications, 1978).

BLAKELEE, SANDRA, 'The Physical Roots of Emotion', *International Herald Tribune* (8 Dec. 1994), 8.

BROCKBANK, NICHOLAS, review of Jonathan Drake, *Body Know-how*, *Alexander Journal*, 12 (autumn 1992), 48–9.

BUNTING, CHRISTOPHER, *Essay on the Craft of Cello-Playing*, vol. ii: *The Left Hand* (Cambridge: Cambridge University Press, 1982).

CARRINGTON, WALTER, *On the Alexander Technique, in Discussion with Séan Carey* (London: Sheildrake Press, 1986).

CHISSELL, JOAN, *Schumann*, 3rd rev. edn. (London: J. M. Dent and Sons Ltd., 1977).

CLUFF, R. A., 'Chronic Hyperventilation and its Treatment by Physiotherapy: Discussion Paper', *Journal of the Royal Society of Medicine*, 77 (Oct. 1984), 855–61.

COGHILL, GEORGE, 'Appreciation', in Alexander, *UCL*, pp. xxi–xxviii.

CONNER, STEVE, 'The Brain Machines', *Independent on Sunday Review* (7 Nov. 1993), 76.

COUSINS, NORMAN, *Anatomy of an Illness as Perceived by the Patient: Reflections on Healing and Regeneration* (New York, Bantam Books, 1981).

DALE, DELBERT A., *Trumpet Technique* (Oxford: Oxford University Press, 1965).

DALTON, DAVID, *Playing the Viola: Conversations with William Primrose* (Oxford: Oxford University Press, 1988).

FENN, WALLACE O., and RAHN, HERMANN, eds., *Handbook of Physiology: A Critical, Comprehensive Presentation of Physiological Knowledge and Concepts, Section 3: Respiration* (Washington, DC: American Physiological Society, 1964).

FOWLER, H. W., *Modern English Usage*, 2nd edn., rev. Ernest Gowers (Oxford: Clarendon Press, 1965, repr. 1968).

Fuchs, Viktor, *The Art of Singing and Voice Technique: A Handbook for Voice Teachers, for Professional and Amateur Singers* (London: Calder & Boyars, 1973).

Furtwängler, Wilhelm, *Notebooks 1924–1954*, trans. Shaun Whiteside, ed. and with an Introduction by Michael Tanner (London: Quartet Books, 1989).

Galamian, Ivan, *Principles of Violin Playing and Teaching*, 2nd edn. (Englewood Cliffs, NJ: Prentice-Hall, 1985).

Gobbi, Tito, with Ida Cook, *My Life* (London: Macdonald and Jane's, 1979).

Goossens, Leon, and Roxburgh, Edwin, *Oboe* (Yehudi Menuhin Music Guides; London and Sydney: Macdonald & Co., 1977).

Hogg, Margaret E., *A Biology of Man*, vol. ii: *Man the Animal* (London: Heinemann Educational Books, 1966).

Horowitz, Joseph, *Conversations with Arrau* (New York: Knopf, 1982).

Husler, Frederick, and Rodd-Marling, Yvonne, *Singing: The Physical Nature of the Vocal Organ. A Guide to the Unlocking of the Singing Voice* (London: Faber and Faber Ltd., 1965).

Jones, Frank Pierce, *Body Awareness in Action: A Study of the Alexander Technique*, with an Introduction by J. McVicker Hunt (New York: Schocken Books, 1976).

Kleist, Heinrich von, 'The Marioniette Theatre', in Nancy Wilson Ross, ed., *The World of Zen* (New York: Vintage Paperbacks, 1960), 293–9.

Lamperti, Giovanni Battista, *Vocal Wisdom: Maxims Transcribed and Edited by William Earl Brown* (New York: Taplinger Publishing Co. Inc., 1931).

Lee, Bruce, *The Tao of Jeet Kune Do* (Burbank, Calif.: Ohara Publications, Inc., 1975).

Lieberman, Julie Lyonn, *You are your Instrument* (New York: Huiski Music, 1991).

Lum, L. C., 'Hyperventilation and Anxiety State', *Journal of the Royal Society of Medicine*, 74 (Jan. 1981), 1–4.

McCallion, Michael, *The Voice Book* (London: Faber and Faber, 1989).

Macdonald, Patrick, 'Six Essentials for a Teacher of the F. Matthias Alexander Technique' (unpublished paper, 10 July 1970).

—— *The Alexander Technique as I See it* (Brighton: Rahula Books, 1989).

Mantel, Gerhard, *Cello Technique: Principles and Forms of Movement*, trans. Barbara Haimberger Thiem (Bloomington, Ind.: Indiana University Press, 1975).

Matheopoulos, Helena, *Maestro: Encounters with Conductors of Today* (London: Hutchinson, 1982).

Matthay, Tobias, *An Epitome of the Laws of Pianoforte Technique, being a Summary Abstracted from 'The Visible and Invisible', a Digest of the Author's Technical Writings* (London: Humphrey Milford, 1931; repr. London: Oxford University Press, 1972).

Mejia, Carlos M. Ramos, *La dinamica del violinista* (Buenos Aires: Ricordi Americana, 1947).

Merrick, Frank, *Practising the Piano* (London: Rockliff, 1958).

Miller, Richard, *English, French, German, and Italian Techniques of Singing: A Study in National Tonal Preferences and how they Relate to Functional Efficiency* (Methuen, NJ: The Scarecrow Press, 1977).

Monsaingeon, Bruno, *Mademoiselle: Conversations with Nadia Boulanger*, trans. Robyn Marsack (Manchester: Carcanet Press, 1985).

Neuhaus, Heinrich, *The Art of Piano Playing*, trans. K. A. Leibovitch (London: Barrie and Jenkins, 1973).

Ogawa, Hiroide, *Enlightenment through the Art of Basketball*, trans. H. Taniguchi, James N. Delavaye, and Otis McCrail, with images by Peter Nuttall (Cambridge and New York: The Oleander Press, 1979).

Pleeth, William, *Cello* (Yehudi Menuhin Music Guides; London and Sydney: Macdonald & Co., 1982).

Reid, Cornelius L., *The Free Voice: A Guide to Natural Singing* (New York: Joseph Patelson Music House, 1972).

—— *A Dictionary of Vocal Terminology: An Analysis* (New York: Joseph Patelson Music House, 1983).

—— *Essays on the Nature of Singing* (Huntsville, Tex.: Recital Publications, 1992).

Rockstro, Richard Shepherd, *A Treatise on the Flute*, 2nd edn. (London: Musica Rara, 1928; repr. 1967).

Running with Style (Mt. View, Calif.: World Publications, 1975).

Sacks, Oliver, *The Man who Mistook his Wife for a Hat and Other Clinical Tales* (New York: Harper Perennial, 1990).

Sandor, Gyorgy, *On Piano Playing: Motion, Sound and Expression* (New York: Schirmer Books, 1981).

Schonberg, Harold C., *The Great Pianists* (London: Victor Gollancz, 1974).

Sherrington, Charles, *The Integrative Action of the Nervous System*, 2nd edn. (New Haven: Yale University Press, 1961).

Starker, Janos, 'An Organized Method of String Playing'. In Murray Grodner, ed., *Concepts in String Playing: Reflections by Artist-Teachers at the Indiana School of Music* (Bloomington, Ind., and London: Indiana University Press, 1979), 133–55.

Stuckenschmidt, H. H., *Ferruccio Busoni: Chronicle of a European*, trans. Sandra Morris (London: Calder & Boyars, 1970).

Toff, Nancy, *The Flute Book* (London: David & Charles, 1985).

Trevelyan, George, 'Training with F. M.', *Alexander Journal*, 12 (autumn 1992), 13–28.

Wanless, Mary, *Ride with your Mind: A Right Brain Approach to Riding* (London: The Kingswood Press, 1991).

WICK, DENIS, *Trombone Technique*, rev. edn. (London: Oxford University Press, 1973).

WILLIAMS, RICHARD, 'Age of the Rocket Man', *Independent on Sunday Review* (20 June 93), 10–11.

WINGATE, PETER, with WINGATE, RICHARD, *The Penguin Medical Encyclopedia*, 3rd edn. (London: Penguin Books, 1988).

Index